IMAGING IN RADIOTHERAPY

Imaging in Radiotherapy

JUDY TAYLOR

CROOM HELM
London & Sydney

© 1988 Judy Taylor
Croom Helm Ltd, Provident House,
Burrell Row, Beckenham, Kent BR3 1AT
Croom Helm Australia, 44-50 Waterloo Road,
North Ryde, 2113, New South Wales

British Library Cataloguing in Publication Data

Taylor, Judy
   Imaging in radiotherapy.
   1. Radiotherapy, Medical   2. Diagnostic
   imaging   3. Image processing
   I. Title
   616.07′572   RC78.7.D53
   ISBN 0-7099-4317-2

Distributed exclusively in the USA by Sheridan House Inc.,
145 Palisade Street, Dobbs Ferry NY 10522

Typeset in 10 point Times by Leaper & Gard Ltd, Bristol
Printed and bound in Great Britain by
Biddles Ltd, Guildford and King's Lynn

Contents

TO MY MOTHER AND FATHER

Foreword

It is a great pleasure to introduce this book to the readers as it has been produced with an enormous amount of self-discipline and commitment by the author.

It is hard to realise that despite the fact that therapy radiographers have been involved with imaging in planning for many years, no book has been specifically written for them before. This book was planned and written for just that purpose.

Therapy radiographers seeking information on this subject have previously had to rely on sections in different books which did not always apply to their situation, or they could turn to their diagnostic counterparts who couldn't always understand their queries! This book now fulfils their needs.

This book will certainly be used by therapy radiographers wishing to know more about imaging from recording media, through equipment to final results, but also, I suspect, by diagnostic radiographers wanting to find out what it really was their therapy colleagues needed to understand about the subject!

Margaret McClellan
TDCR DPHE
Principal (Co-ordinator)
Schools of Radiography (Diagnosis and Therapy)
Middlesex and University College Hospitals
London

Preface

Realising that many therapy radiographers know little about imaging, and that it is an important part of radiotherapy planning, I decided to write this book for my profession. I hope it will be useful for students, radiographers studying for higher qualifications and anyone with an interest in radiotherapy planning.

I would especially like to thank the following for all their generous help and advice: O. Deaville, Dr Delpy, S. Hay, M. Lovegrove, M. McClellan, M. Robinson, J. Stock, B. Turner and M. Viljoen.

I must also thank all the staff at the Middlesex and University College Hospitals Schools of Radiography (Diagnosis and Therapy) for their patience, and everyone who has helped with the artwork, in particular those who sent slides or photographs, or gave permission for me to reproduce their diagrams.

Many thanks to Dr Spittle, who allowed me to use her computer, without which I would not have attempted the book; and to Teresa Young, who spent much time helping me to understand how this computer functioned.

J.T.

1

The Structure of X-ray Film

Manufacturers of X-ray film all have their own trade secrets, but the basic structure of the film is the same. It consists of a sensitive emulsion coated on one or both sides of a base.

FILM BASE

The film base is made from polyester and is the thickest layer in the structure of an X-ray film. It is 0.18 mm thick[1] and the whole X-ray film from 0.2 to 0.38 mm in thickness. Some manufacturers make the base by rolling a heated synthetic resin and plasticiser mixture.[2] This is formed into thin sheets which are stretched and dried, and then put onto large spools. The base material must be stored in a dust-free environment until it is needed for coating with the emulsion.

Properties of the film base

To transmit light

This ensures the sensitive emulsion receives as much light as possible to produce the latent image (see Chapter 4). A blue tint is given to the base, as this reduces the glare when viewing the final image with an illuminator (see Chapter 4), and the eye is more perceptive to the blue colour. However, the blue tint affects the ability of the base to transmit light and there is slightly more basic fog on the film (see Chapter 3). A blue-based film has a density of 0.15 whereas a clear-based film has a density of 0.10 (see Chapter 3). Traditionally the blue-based films are preferred.

To be flexible, strong and tear resistant

The strength of the base is very important as it acts as a support for all the other layers; it must also withstand handling by automatic processors.

Non-flammable

The base has to be a 'safety base', in other words it must not be prone to spontaneous combustion.

To be of uniform thickness and free from defects

A regular thickness of the base is required with no defects, so that it can be evenly coated with the emulsion.

Chemically inactive

For stability the base must be impermeable to water and the chemicals used during processing.

SUBBING LAYER (SUBSTRATUM)

The subbing layer acts as an adhesive bonding the emulsion to the base of the X-ray film. It is made of synthetic resins and is on both sides of the base.

EMULSION

The photosensitive layer is the emulsion, and it consists of silver halide crystals suspended in gelatin. On exposure to visible light, X-rays or gamma rays this layer changes structurally to form a latent image, and when processed a visible image (see Chapter 4).

Silver halides

The silver halides, silver bromide, silver chloride and silver iodide, are produced by mixing a solution of silver nitrate with a solution of a potassium halide.

$$AgNO_3 + KX = AgX + KNO_3$$
Silver nitrate + potassium halide = silver halide + potassium nitrate

The silver halides are in the form of tiny crystals or grains, generally pebble-shaped or globular. If the crystals are produced with a flattened surface, known as tabular or 'T' grain, facing towards the image source, the crystals will absorb more electromagnetic radiation which is needed to produce the latent image.

Silver bromide is used as the main constituent of the emulsion with approximately 2 per cent silver iodide to help obtain the correct speed for the film. Silver chloride could be used as it has rapid development and fixing properties, but the disadvantage is that it has a lower photosensitivity than silver bromide.[1]

Gelatin

Gelatin is used so that the silver halide crystals are evenly distributed throughout the emulsion and do not clump together. It has impurities added, such as sulphur to help latent image formation. The gelatin also protects the latent image in the time interval between exposure to radiation and processing of the film. It does this by not allowing the halide ions to recombine with the silver, as this would destroy the latent image.

The gelatin sets firmly after coating on to the base but still gives flexibility. A disadvantage of gelatin is that when it is placed in a warm solution, for example during processing, it will soften. To help prevent this, hardeners can be added to the gelatin. It must be inert to the chemicals which are added during manufacture of the emulsion.

Manufacture of the emulsion

The emulsion is manufactured in total darkness because of the sensitivity of the silver halides to light. Some manufacturers use light-tight tanks in brightly lit rooms. The following processes are carried out during the manufacture.[1-3]

Mixing

An excess of potassium bromide is mixed with the gelatin, and is added to the silver nitrate in a large stainless-steel vat.

Ripening

The solution is stirred at a set temperature for a certain length of time; this allows for an increase in grain size. In general larger grains give greater film speed, a wide range of grain sizes gives low contrast and a narrow range of grain sizes high contrast (see Chapter 3).

Extra gelatin is added, the emulsion is cooled by placing the vat in ice water and a jelly-like substance is formed. This is then shredded and washed in pure water to remove the by-product of potassium nitrate and any remaining potassium bromide, so the silver halide and gelatin are left behind as the emulsion.

Digestion

The shredded emulsion is remelted and maintained at a constant temperature. Various sensitisers can be added at this stage to increase the sensitivity (speed) of the emulsion.

Other additives

After sufficient digestion has taken place more substances can be added to the emulsion to extend the colour sensitivity, and to improve the physical characteristics of the film.

Silver halides are naturally sensitive to ultraviolet light and the blue region of the spectrum and less sensitive to X and gamma radiation.

For monochromatic emulsion

There is no addition of colour sensitisers and the film is sensitive to the blue region of the spectrum and ultraviolet light.

For orthochromatic emulsion

The addition of colour sensitisers, in the form of dyes, is necessary, and this gives sensitivity to the blue region plus the green and yellow regions of the spectrum.

This is important for matching the spectral sensitivity of the film to the light emission of intensifying screens (see Chapter 2).

To improve the physical characteristics of the film the following substances are added:

(1) *Hardener.* Alum salts make the emulsion tough and resistant to damage during handling and processing.
(2) *Wetting agent.* This helps the gelatin absorb water and wet the emulsion evenly, to allow development to take place and help speed up processing time.
(3) *Bactericide and fungicide.* Prevents the growth of bacteria and mould.
(4) *Plasticiser.* Stops the emulsion becoming too brittle.
(5) *Anti-foggant.* This keeps the basic fog level to a minimum (see Chapter 3).
(6) *Anti-frothing agent.* Helps prevent bubbles forming during coating.

For a summary of this process see Figure 1.1.

Figure 1.1: Manufacture of the emulsion.

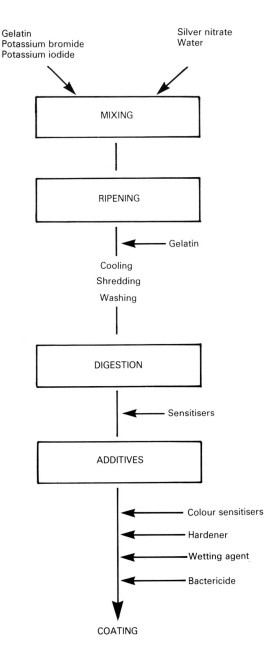

Figure 1.2: The structure of single-sided X-ray film.

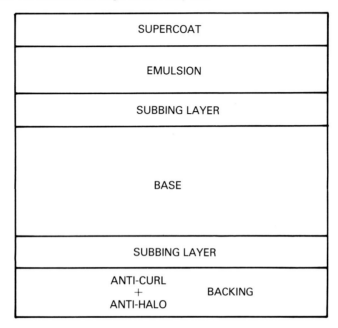

COATING OF THE EMULSION

The technique of emulsion coating is very specialised and complex. The emulsion layer must be evenly spread over the whole area of the film to give a uniform sensitivity.

Single-sided film

The emulsion is coated on one side of the base (see Figure 1.2). The anti-curl backing is necessary, because without it the emulsion will shrink and curl inwards when dried during processing. The backing is made up of a layer of gelatin the same thickness as the emulsion. The anti-halo backing is needed because of the reflection of light at the base when the film is exposed to radiation. This causes a halo or fogging of the image (see Figure 1.3a). A dark-coloured dye is added to the gelatin of the anti-curl backing to help prevent this fogging by absorbing the reflected light (see Figure 1.3b). The dye must be bleached out during processing so that the image can be viewed. The anti-curl and the anti-halo backing therefore become one layer. Single-sided film is used for:

(1) Mammography

(2) Monitor photography — computed tomography, ultrasound and radio-nuclide imaging
(3) Fluorography — photography of an image on a fluorescent screen
(4) Copying radiographs
(5) Subtraction — a special imaging technique to show the outline of vessels rather than bones and soft tissue

A disadvantage of single-sided film is that the emulsion must be placed towards the source which will irradiate it. Therefore it is always necessary to put the film the correct way round in the cassette. The emulsion layer is a pale colour in daylight conditions but the film must not be exposed in this manner or it will become fogged and useless. The emulsion generally has a matt surface which can be seen under safe-light conditions in the darkroom, and the opposite side is shiny. Manufacturers put a notch on one edge of the film, so that when it is felt in the top right-hand corner the emulsion is towards the viewer.[4, 5]

Duplitised film (double-sided film)

Duplitised films are used for general radiography. The emulsion is coated on both sides of the base (see Figure 1.4). The anti-curl layer is not needed because the emulsion will shrink equally on both sides when dried during

Figure 1.3a: Halation in a single-sided film without anti-halation layer. (Reproduced by permission of David Jenkins and MTP Press Ltd.)

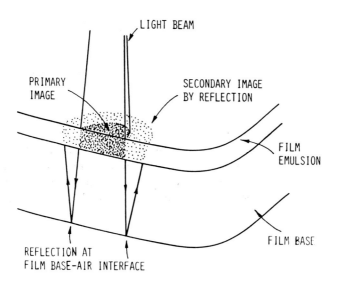

Figure 1.3b: Prevention of halation in a single-sided film. (Reproduced by permission of David Jenkins and MTP Press Ltd.)

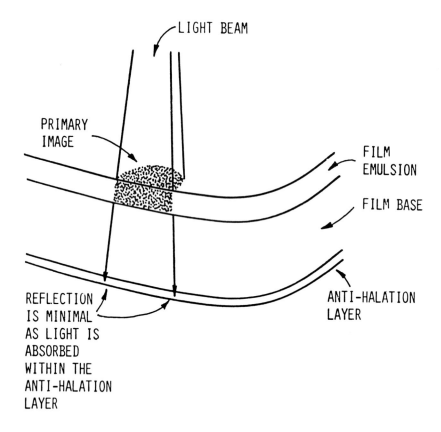

processing. There is no anti-halo backing. Film handling is easy as it does not matter which way round duplitised film is loaded into the cassette.

SUPERCOAT

The supercoat is a thin layer of gelatin over the emulsion layer. It protects the sensitive emulsion from damage and provides a smooth surface that is less likely to attract dirt and dust. The supercoat is the final coat, and the film is now a finished product. It is cut into suitable sizes, stored and eventually distributed.

Figure 1.4: The structure of double-sided (duplitised) X-ray film.

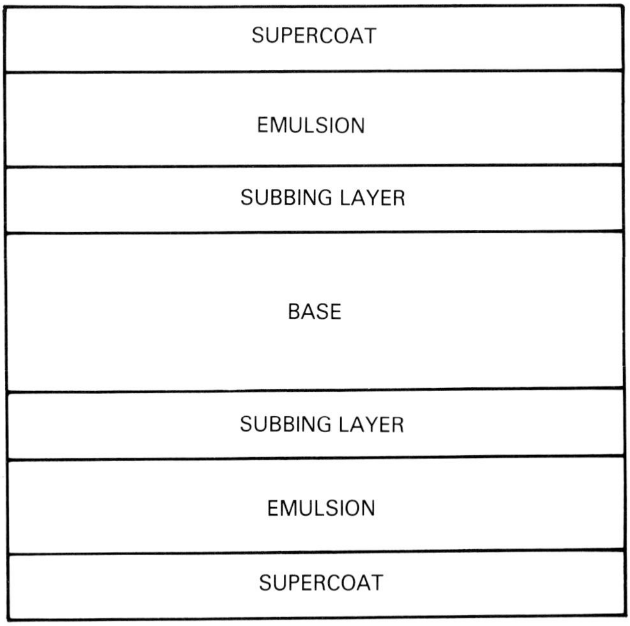

SUPERCOAT
EMULSION
SUBBING LAYER
BASE
SUBBING LAYER
EMULSION
SUPERCOAT

TYPES OF FILM USED IN RADIOTHERAPY

Screen-type film

Screen-type films are used with intensifying screens (see Chapter 2) and are sensitive to different wavelengths of light depending on the colour sensitisers in their emulsion. This is referred to as the spectral sensitivity of the film. Blue- or green-sensitive duplitised films are used for localisation with a simulator (see Chapter 6). It is important that the film matches the light emission of the intensifying screen. Exposures can be given using the simulator so that the images produced have good definition (see Chapter 3).

This imaging system, of films with intensifying screens, unfortunately cannot be used effectively for verification with the high-energy radiotherapy equipment. This is because only a small amount of the penetrating radiation is absorbed in the emulsion of the film, and an acceptable image is not produced. However some radiotherapy departments try to overcome this problem by using lead or copper screens with screen-type films, as explained in Chapter 2. The most commonly used sizes of films are:

9

18 cm × 24 cm
24 cm × 30 cm   10″ × 12″
30 cm × 40 cm
35 cm × 35 cm
35 cm × 43 cm   14″ × 17″

Cost depends on the type and size of film; prices range from 30p to £1.50 a sheet (1985/6 prices).

Direct exposure film

This film is used without intensifying screens and is directly exposed to the radiation to form an image. It is used in radiotherapy for verifying treatment areas on the treatment units, which range from a 250 kV set to a 16 MV linear accelerator. This immediately poses a problem for the film as it must have a wide latitude (see Chapter 3) to encompass the range of energy, and at the higher energies contrast between bone and soft tissue diminishes. The film needs a slow speed (see Chapter 3) and a thicker emulsion than for screen-type films.

Industrial film

This is a direct exposure film which is suitable for verification. The disadvantage is that this film must either be manually processed, or have a cycle time in an automatic processor of between three and eight minutes. The cost varies from 45p to £2.55 a sheet, depending on size and packing (1985/6 prices).

However, there are two different kinds of direct exposure film which can be automatically processed in the shorter 90-second cycle, and these at present are only produced by Eastman Kodak Company. These are the X-OMAT V and X-OMAT TL films, which are separately packed in light-tight envelopes. Prices range from £1.50 to £3.00 a sheet, depending on the size required.

(1) *X-OMAT V film.* This can be left underneath the patient throughout the whole treatment time (see Figure 1.5a). The film has a very slow speed, about twelve times slower than the other Kodak direct exposure film. The advantage of this film is that the patient is not moved during the procedure. There is one slight disadvantage: as only the treatment area is seen on the viewed film, especially if it is a small area, it can be difficult to orientate.

(2) *X-OMAT TL film.* This film can be used for localisation with a simulator (see Chapter 6) and for verification on the treatment unit. For verification purposes the film must be removed after a short exposure and cannot remain in position for the duration of the treatment. A

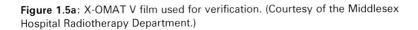

Figure 1.5a: X-OMAT V film used for verification. (Courtesy of the Middlesex Hospital Radiotherapy Department.)

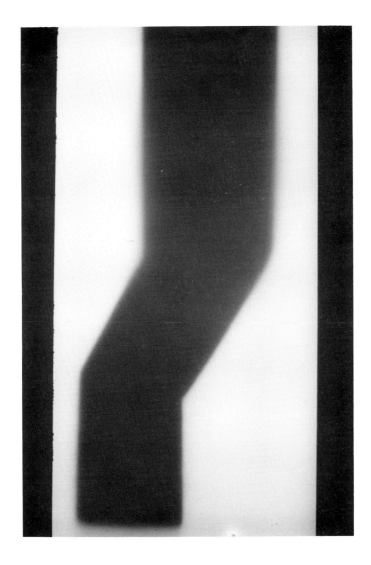

Figure 1.5b: X-OMAT TL film used for verification (double exposure). (Courtesy of the Middlesex Hospital Radiotherapy Department.)

double or single exposure can be given depending on the field size of the treatment area.

For a small volume the field size is opened out, so that bony landmarks can be seen when the film is viewed and are therefore easier to orientate. This larger area is given an exposure of 3–5 cGy (or equivalent in monitor units) and then the field size returned to the correct setting for the patient and another exposure of 3–5 cGy given (see Figure 1.5b). The film is then removed and patients must have their treatment area checked to make sure they are still in the correct position. For larger field sizes a single exposure can be given of 6–10 cGy, and once again the film is removed and the area rechecked so treatment can continue. This is of course a disadvantage as it disturbs the patient and the treatment area, and takes longer than just leaving the film under the patient for the treatment time. To find the most useful exposure on the different treatment machines, head-and-body phantoms can be used to simulate the patient.

Better contrast can be seen with this film than the other Kodak direct exposure film, especially if lead or copper screens are used (see Chapter 2), either in a cassette or a light-tight film holder.

Some departments use screen-type film with lead screens, instead of the direct exposure film, for verification on the treatment unit. The lead screens are from 0.1 to 0.5 mm thick, placed on both sides of the film. The film shows good definition and has the advantage of being slightly cheaper to purchase than the direct exposure film.

XERORADIOGRAPHS

Xeroradiography is the recording of an image on a charged plate. This system can be used for localisation on the simulator and for verification on the treatment unit.[6-9]

The Xerox plate is 35 × 25 cm, made of aluminium, coated with a very fine layer of selenium, and when ready for use is contained in a light-tight plastic cassette. The selenium is an insulator in the dark, but when exposed to light it becomes more conductive and this helps form a latent image on the plate. When the plate is charged and exposed to radiation the area irradiated will be more conductive and lose charge, and the unexposed areas will remain charged. Thus an image is formed on the plate by the electric charges and the uncharged areas. An automated system is used to charge the plate and also to develop the image.

Xerox System 125

This consists of the conditioner and processor, each approximately 1m high, 1 m in depth and 0.5 m in width. These two units can be placed in a well-ventilated space and need 240 volt mains power supply. Darkroom facilities are not required (see Figure 1.6).

Figure 1.6: The processor (left) and conditioner (right). (Reproduced by permission of the Middlesex and University College Hospitals Schools of Radiography, Therapy and Diagnosis.)

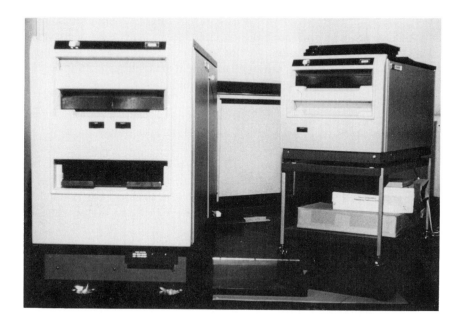

The conditioner

A storage box containing up to six plates is put into the conditioner (see Figure 1.7, 1). The selenium surface is relaxed, which means that all residual charges are removed as the plates are passed through the oven. These plates are stored in a chamber in the conditioner until ready for use. When the empty cassette is inserted into the conditioner one plate is immediately retrieved from storage and passed beneath an air ionisation device so that a positive electric charge is placed on the plate (see Figure 1.7, 3). Varying the amount of charge will slightly change the contrast of the final image (see Figure 1.7, 2); a small thin object needs a less charged plate. The plate is then loaded into the light-tight cassette automatically (see Figure 1.7, 3).

14

Figure 1.7: The Xerox System 125. (Reproduced by permission of Xerox Medical Systems International.)

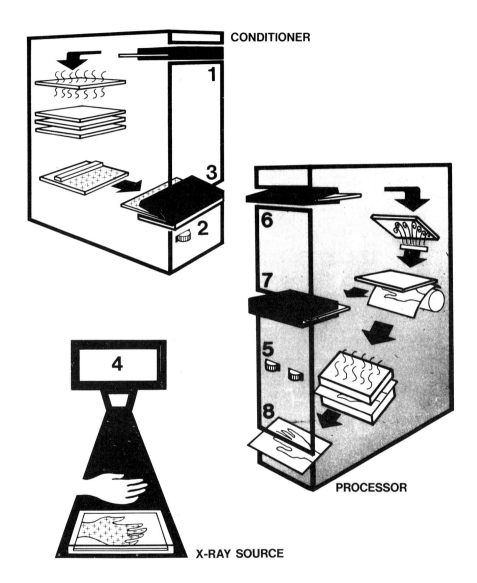

Use — exposure

The Xerox plate when charged in its cassette is used in the same way as a cassette containing intensifying screens, and the appropriate X-ray film (see Figure 1.7, 4). A xeroradiograph taken with a simulator or with diag-

15

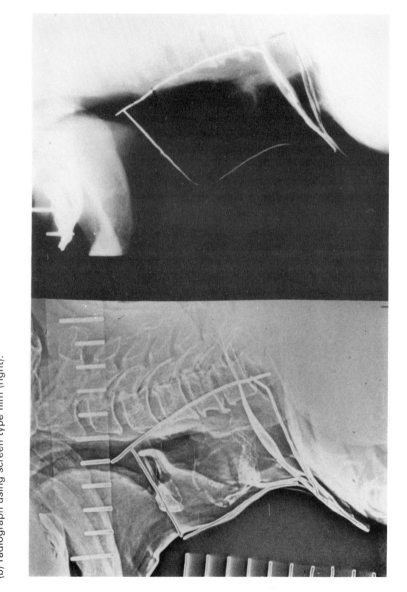

Figure 1.8: Localisation of the larynx using a simulator. (Reproduced by permission of N.J. Noscoe, Middlesex Hospital Medical School.) (a) Xeroradiograph (left); (b) radiograph using screen-type film (right).

Figure 1.9: Verification of the treatment area for a pituitary tumour, using a linear accelerator. (Reproduced by permission of N.J. Noscoe, Middlesex Hospital Medical School.) (a) Xeroradiograph (left); (b) radiograph using direct exposure film (right).

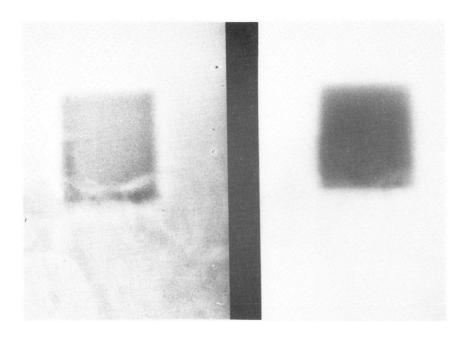

nostic equipment, to image head and neck structures, is given an exposure of 120 kV and 32–40 mAs. To show a similar image using screen-type film an exposure of 140 kV and 2–4 mAs (see Chapter 6, General Guide to Exposure Factors) can be used, and therefore more incident radiation is required for the xeroradiograph.

The xeroradiograph has a wide recording latitude, which means it can image soft tissue and bones, and give good definition to both with the same exposure (see Figure 1.8). It has a slower speed than screen-type film but is faster than direct exposure film. Because of its slower speed it is useful for verification on the treatment units. A dose of 4 cGy will produce a reasonable image (see Figure 1.9), especially in the head and neck region. Unfortunately the pelvic and abdomen areas do not image so well. Another disadvantage to this procedure is that the Xerox plate is pressure-sensitive so the patient would not be able to lie directly on top of the Xerox cassette; a special insert in the treatment couch would be needed. The pressure would cause the selenium to come into contact with the cassette and therefore a discharge would take place and no latent image could be formed.[7]

The processor

After the plate has been exposed to radiation it is inserted into the processor still in its cassette. The plate is unloaded automatically from the cassette in the processor and then passed to the development chamber (see Figure 1.7, 6). A fine blue powder (toner) is blown over the plate. The powder is charged by friction with equal numbers of positive and negative charges.

A choice can be made as to whether a positive or negative image is required (see Figure 1.7, 5). The negative image shows the skeleton in lighter tones and the positive is the opposite, with the skeleton in darker tones. For radiotherapy localisation and verification, negative images are preferred; a positive image is normally used in mammography.

The plate is now automatically moved so it makes contact with the plasticised paper which is already stored in the processor. An electrostatic charge is placed on the back of the paper and the powder from the plate is attracted to the paper. The paper then moves through an oven so that the powder fuses permanently to the paper. The xeroradiograph (as a mirror-image of the original area exposed to radiation) is ready and comes out dry into a tray on the side of the processor (see Figure 1.7, 8). The time taken for development is approximately 90 seconds.

Meanwhile the plate left behind in the processor is cleaned by a rotating brush which removes any remaining powder. The plate is then automatically returned to a storage box (see Figure 1.7, 7). When this box is full it can be re-inserted into the conditioner and the plates can be used again.

Viewing the xeroradiograph

The finished image is on plasticised paper in blue and white tones. It can be viewed adequately in a bright room; no viewing box or special illuminator is needed.

Summary of advantages

(1) Striking contrast of image
(2) No viewer necessary
(3) No darkroom or plumbing requirements for water supply (see Chapter 4)
(4) Wide recording latitude
(5) No grid required as less sensitive to scatter (see Chapter 2)
(6) Re-usable plate

Summary of disadvantages

(1) Expensive; approximate prices of equipment shown below (1985/6 prices):

    Cassette — £257
    One plate — £185
    500 sheets of paper — £145
    One bottle of toner — £59.50
    Cost to rent units — £483 per month
    Cost to buy units — £41,000

(2) Pressure-sensitive

(3) Handling problems — plate must be used immediately after being charged and processed straight after exposure, or charge will leak and latent image fades

(4) More exposure required than for screen-type film

REFERENCES

1. Kodak, 'X-ray recording materials', *Fundamentals of Radiographic Photography*, vol. II, pp. 3–10.
2. Fuji, 'Fundamentals of sensitised materials for radiography', *Fuji Film Technical Handbook*, pp. 4–7.
3. Agfa Gevaert, *The Manufacture of Film*, Technical literature.
4. Chesney, D.N. and Chesney, M.O. (1981) *Radiographic Imaging*, 4th edn, Blackwell Scientific Publications, Oxford, pp. 14–49.
5. Jenkins, D. (1980) *Radiographic Photography and Imaging Processes*, MTP Press, Lancaster, pp. 8–13.
6. Meredith, W.J. and Massey, J.B. (1977) *Fundamental Physics of Radiology*, 3rd edn, Wright, Bristol, pp. 205–10.
7. Noscoe, N.J. (1980) 'Xerotomography of the larynx — an aid to radiotherapy planning', *Radiography*, September, pp. 199–205.
8. Chesney, D.N. and Chesney, M.O. (1981) *Radiographic Imaging*, 4th edn, Blackwell Scientific Publications, Oxford, pp. 491–7.
9. Jenkins, D. (1980) *Radiographic Photography and Imaging Processes*, MTP Press, Lancaster, pp. 266–70.

Private communications

T. Cropper (Marketing Education Centre, Kodak); K. Jones; N.J. Noscoe; M. Robinson; N. Smith (Agfa Gevaert); J. Stock; B. Turner; M. Webster.

Manufacturers' literature

Agfa Gevaert, 'Diagnostic Imaging Systems Medical Division Price List', April 1985.

Kodak, 'Medical Buyers Guide to the DHSS', April 1985.
3M, Diagnostic Imaging Systems, Product Directory.
3M, XUD Ultra detail X-ray Film.
Xerox Medical Systems International, Xerox for Xeroradiography, 125 System.

FURTHER READING

Gifford, D. (1984) *A Handbook of Physics for Radiologists and Radiographers*, John Wiley and Sons, Chichester, pp. 196–203.

2

Screens, Cassettes and Grids

X-RAY INTENSIFYING SCREENS

The use of intensifying screens with X-ray film has enabled the amount of radiation needed for the exposure (see Chapters 3 and 5) to be reduced, without affecting image quality. The screens amplify the effects of the radiation reaching the film, and so less incident radiation is required.

Principles of intensifying screens

The intensifying screens absorb radiation which is converted into many light photons, and this light exposes the emulsion of the X-ray film to produce a latent image (see Chapter 4). The screens are able to do this because they contain a phosphor layer.[1]

Phosphor

This substance is luminescent and emits light photons when irradiated by X-rays, gamma rays or ultraviolet light. It involves two processes: fluorescence and phosphorescence.[2,3]

Fluorescence

The light photons are emitted while the phosphor is irradiated, but stop almost immediately when the radiation ceases.

Phosphorescence

This effect is sometimes called 'afterglow' because the light photons continue to be emitted from the phosphor after the incident radiation has stopped. Phosphorescence needs to be reduced when using intensifying screens, and is controlled by adding impurities, called 'killers', into the phosphor.

Figure 2.1: The structure of an intensifying screen. (Reproduced by permission of Kodak Ltd.)

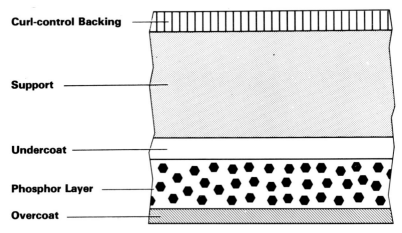

Curl-control Backing

Support

Undercoat

Phosphor Layer

Overcoat

STRUCTURE OF THE X-RAY INTENSIFYING SCREEN

A diagram of the structure of the intensifying screen is shown in Figure 2.1.

Support-base

The support or base is made of polyester or cardboard and is strong and flexible. It has to be chemically inert so that it does not react with the phosphor layer. It is moisture-resistant and has a backing layer to prevent the screen curling.

Undercoat

The undercoat provides a close contact between the support and phosphor layer and acts as a bonding layer. If it contains a white pigment, such as titanium dioxide, the undercoat also acts as a reflector layer.[4] It reflects light photons back towards the emulsion which otherwise would have been lost through the screen (see Figure 2.2a). Unfortunately the light does not reflect back exactly in the direction of the original light, and causes a slight spreading of the beam which will blur the final image (see Figure 2.2b).

Phosphor layer

The phosphor layer has a uniform coating of tiny phosphor crystals

Figure 2.2a: Intensifying screen without reflector layer. (Reproduced by permission of Kodak Ltd.)

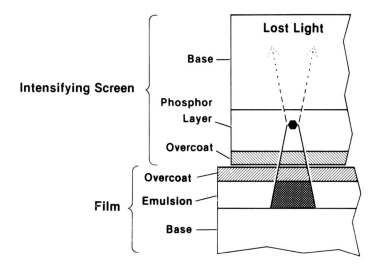

Figure 2.2b: Intensifying screen with reflector layer. (Reproduced by permission of Kodak Ltd.)

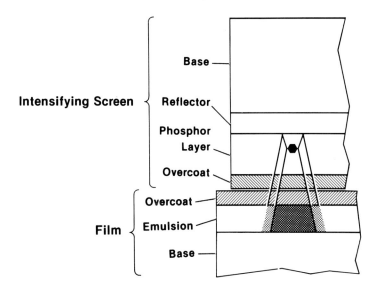

suspended in polyurethane, cellulose or nylon. Light photons are emitted from the phosphor crystals in all directions, which will make the image slightly blurred (see Chapter 3). To prevent this, carbon granules or a dye can be added to the phosphor layer to absorb some of the sideways spread of the light photons; this will, however, reduce the speed of the screen.

The amount of phosphor material per unit area of the screen is called the coating weight, and depends on the size of the phosphor crystal and thickness of the phosphor layer. In practice the phosphor crystals are generally of the same size but the thickness of the layer is varied. A thick layer of phosphor material will allow more light photons to be emitted than will a thin layer, but it will slightly blur the image as the light photons will be able to spread out further before reaching the emulsion of the film.[4]

Most phosphors require an activator to make them more efficient at producing light photons. The activator is an impurity added to the phosphor, and it alters the atomic structure of the material to improve its luminescent qualities.

There are many different types of phosphors but only the ones that absorb X-rays efficiently, strongly fluoresce and have little phosphorescence are useful in X-ray intensifying screens. Some of the phosphors used are mentioned below.

Calcium tungstate

This phosphor is common for conventional screens, and the emission of the light photons are in the blue and ultraviolet region of the spectrum.

Barium fluorochloride

This is activated with europium and emits blue and ultraviolet light. It is more efficient at absorbing radiation and converting it into light photons than is calcium tungstate, and requires about half the amount of radiation for the same density image (see Chapter 3).

Rare earth phosphors

These are a group of soft malleable metals. Some of the different types being used in intensifying screens are listed below.

Lanthanum oxybromide emits blue light.
Yttrium oxysulphide emits blue light.
Gadolinium oxysulphide emits green light.
Lanthanum oxysulphide emits green light.

They are all activated with terbium, which is also a rare earth.

The rare earth phosphors have made intensifying screens even more efficient, and less radiation is needed to produce an image than for the conventional calcium tungstate screens (see Figure 2.3).

Useful energies for producing images for localisation (see Chapter 6) are between 50 and 75 keV, and at these energies rare earth screens are four to five times better at absorbing X-rays than the calcium tungstate screens (see Figure 2.4). Rare earth screens also have a much greater light conversion efficiency — that is, the fraction of incident energy converted into luminescence is 13–18 per cent, whereas with calcium tungstate screens the light conversion efficiency is 3–5 per cent. This means for the same amount of radiation absorbed the rare earth screens will emit more light photons than the calcium tungstate screens.[5]

Overcoat (supercoat)

The overcoat is the protective top layer of the intensifying screen. It is lacquered so that it is scratch-proof and prevents damage occurring to the sensitive phosphor layer when the screen is cleaned (see later in this chapter).

USE OF INTENSIFYING SCREENS

The intensifying screens are mounted into a cassette (see later in this chapter) and used in conjunction with an X-ray film.

With duplitised X-ray film

Details of duplitised film can be found in Chapter 1. When using duplitised film it is necessary to have a front and a back intensifying screen around the film (see Figure 2.5).

When the front and back intensifying screens are irradiated they will emit light and expose the emulsion layer nearest to each screen. Some of

Figure 2.3: Less radiation needed when using rare earth screens. (Reproduced by permission of 3M United Kingdom PLC.)

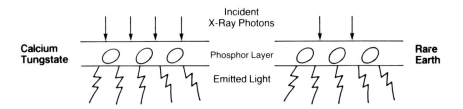

Figure 2.4: $CaWO_4$ = calcium tungstate; LaOBr = lanthanum oxybromide; Gd_2O_2S = gadolinium oxysulphide. (Reproduced by permission of 3M United Kingdom PLC.)

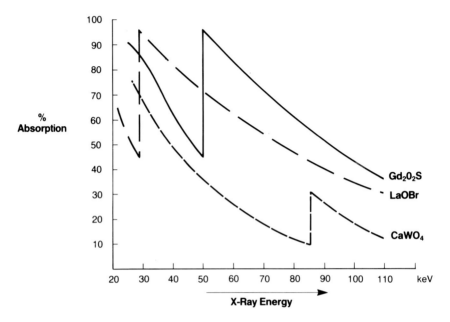

the light is not fully absorbed in that emulsion layer, carries on through the base of the film to expose the opposite emulsion and produces an image. This is the 'cross-over' effect, and a disadvantage of 'cross-over' is that as the light beam passes through the base it spreads out and the image produced in the opposite emulsion is slightly blurred (see Figure 2.6). However an advantage of 'cross-over' is the increase of light producing the image.[4]

Another disadvantage of using intensifying screens is that when the light photons hit the emulsion of the film they are scattered in all directions and cause slight blurring of the image. This is secondary irradiation, and happens because the light photons are reflected off the surface of the silver halide crystals in the emulsion.

With single-sided film

Details of single-sided film can be found in Chapter 1. An intensifying screen is only used with this kind of film when it is exposed to X-rays, for example during mammography. Single-sided film does not need an intensifying screen when it is exposed to light photons as for monitor photography (see Chapter 7). There is only one emulsion layer and the intensifying

Figure 2.5: Front and back intensifying screens with duplitised film. (Reproduced by permission of Kodak Ltd.)

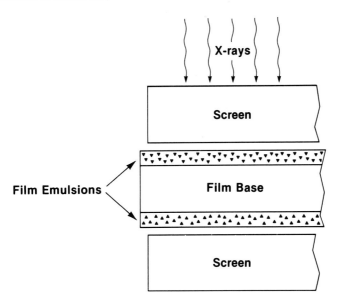

Figure 2.6: To show 'crossover' with intensifying screens. (Reproduced by permission of Kodak Ltd.)

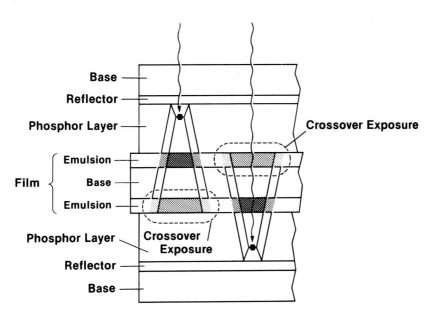

screen is placed underneath the film. It is therefore a back screen with the emulsion nearest to the screen.

The radiation passes through the film to the screen which will emit light photons to produce an image. If the screen were placed on top of the film the radiation would pass through the screen, produce light photons in the upper part of the phosphor layer, and the light photons would spread out before they reach the emulsion. This would cause slightly more blurring of the image than if the screen is beneath the film.[6]

USE OF INTENSIFYING SCREENS IN RADIOTHERAPY

Intensifying screens are used with screen-type film (see Chapter 1) to produce images for localisation of the treatment area with the simulator, a mobile X-ray unit and even a DXR unit (radiotherapy treatment set). To give maximum efficiency the emulsion of the film used should be sensitive to the light emitted by the phosphor of the intensifying screen (see Figures 2.7a and 2.7b).

A screen which emits light photons in the blue part of the spectrum, such as calcium tungstate or the rare earth lanthanum oxybromide, should be used with an X-ray film which is sensitive to blue light. This kind of film is called a monochromatic film (see Chapter 1). For a screen which emits light photons in the green part of the spectrum, gadolinium oxysulphide, an orthochromatic film (see Chapter 1) should be used, which is sensitive to green light.

Sometimes it is necessary to use a film screen combination which is not so efficient. In one radiotherapy department, where only a DXR unit (125 kV) is available for localisation, even on the smallest time setting available the intensity of the radiation is such that a useful image is not produced with the usual film screen combination. To make the imaging system less sensitive to the radiation, and the resources available to that department, a green-sensitive film and a blue-emitting screen were used.

To prove this combination was the most useful in the given circumstances, a green-sensitive film and blue-sensitive film were cut into two and each half placed in the cassette with the blue-emitting screen. The outside of the cassette was marked when loaded with the different films in the darkroom, and identification markers were put on the outside of the cassette. Using this cassette with a secondary radiation grid (see later in this chapter), an image was taken of a head phantom and the films were processed. It could be clearly seen that the green-sensitive film gave a better image than the blue-sensitive film.

Another suitable film in this situation, using the DXR unit for localisation, is the direct exposure film; however, as already mentioned in Chapter 1, this film is more expensive than the screen-type film.

Figure 2.7a: Monochromatic film with appropriate intensifying screen. (Reproduced by permission of Kodak Ltd.)

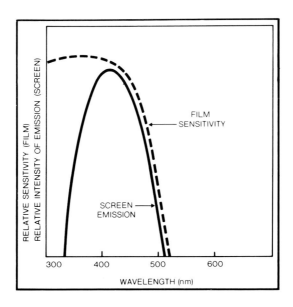

Figure 2.7b: Orthochromatic film with appropriate intensifying screen. (Reproduced by permission of Kodak Ltd.)

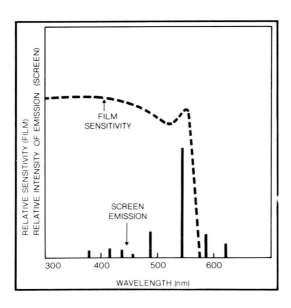

Lead screens

Lead screens are useful when trying to image with high-energy radio-therapy equipment. Good results have been obtained by using screen-type film, or direct exposure film, in between lead screens for verification of a treatment area on the radiotherapy treatment set.

The lead screens are made up of lead sheet with thicknesses ranging from 0.1 to 0.5 mm. They are used in pairs and mounted either in a screen-type cassette, with the intensifying screens removed, or a plastic light-tight holder (see later in this chapter).

The action of the lead is that it absorbs the incident radiation and causes electrons to be ejected, which will produce a latent image (see Chapter 4). It also acts as a filter by reducing the amount of scattered radiation, which will help give a less blurred image. Initial high energy is necessary so that the electrons produced are able to leave the screen and reach the emulsion of the film.

Copper screens

Research at Addenbrookes Radiotherapy department, Cambridge,[7] has recently shown that copper screens are as effective as, if not better than, lead screens, when used in the same way. The X-OMAT TL film (Kodak) used in a Cronex cassette (Du Pont) with a 3 mm copper screen on either side of the film has proved an acceptable combination with a double-exposure technique (see Chapter 1).

Kodak have also produced a new imaging cassette (at present only marketed in the USA) with a copper screen for verification on the treatment unit. The X-OMAT G screen-type film, or X-OMAT V direct exposure film can be used, with different combinations of screens, in the cassette. Depending on which type of film is used, the structure of the back screen is slightly different (for screen-type film see Figure 2.8a and for direct exposure film see Figure 2.8b).

The advantage of using copper is that it is more durable than lead, less easily damaged and gives good film–screen contact.

FILM–SCREEN CONTACT

It is necessary for a good-quality image to have as close a contact between film and screen as possible (see Figure 2.9). The diagram shows that when there is space between the film and screen the divergence of the light photons is greater then when there is no space. This spreading of the beam will create more blurring of the image.

Figure 2.8a: Combination of screens used in therapy cassette for screen-type film. (Reproduced by permission of Kodak Ltd.)

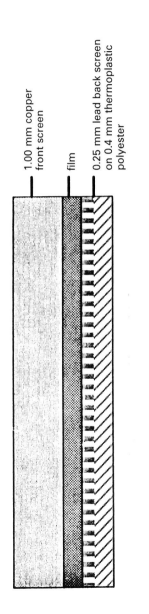

1.00 mm copper front screen

film

0.25 mm lead back screen on 0.4 mm thermoplastic polyester

Figure 2.8b: Combination of screens used in therapy cassette for direct exposure film. (Reproduced by permission of Kodak Ltd.)

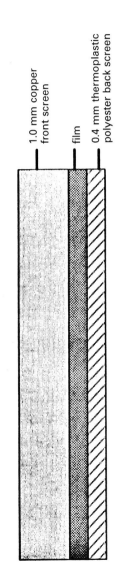

1.0 mm copper front screen

film

0.4 mm thermoplastic polyester back screen

Figure 2.9: Image degradation when there is poor film–screen contact. (Reproduced by permission of Kodak Ltd.)

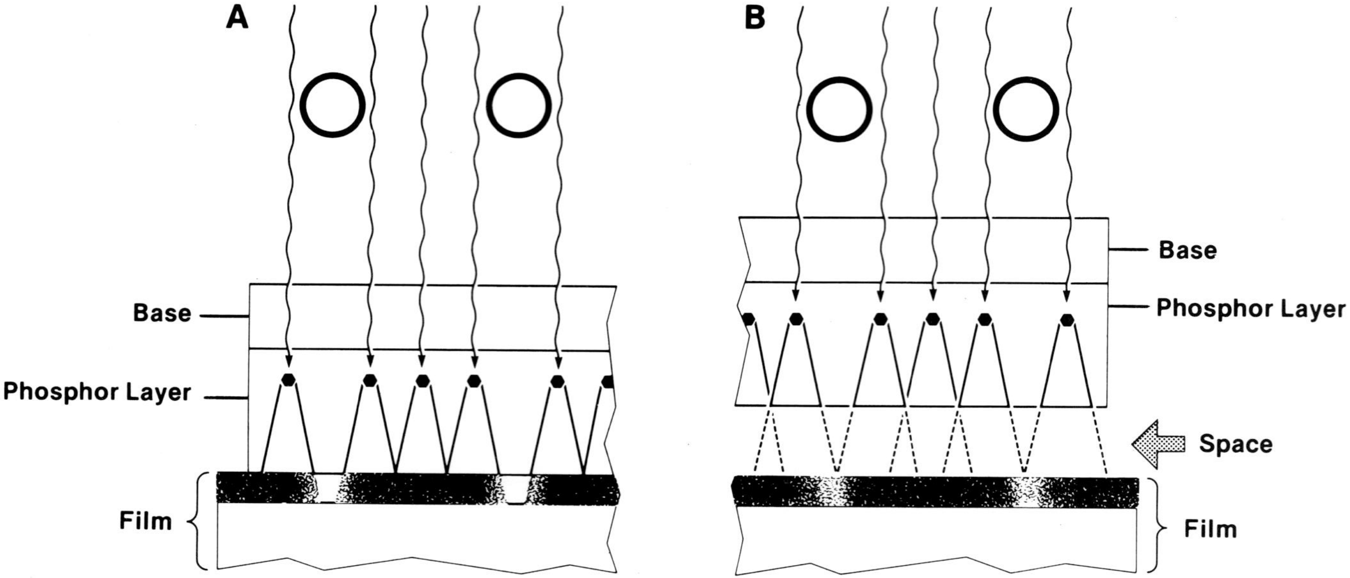

Figure 2.10: Film–screen contact test tool. (Courtesy of Vinten Instruments Ltd.)

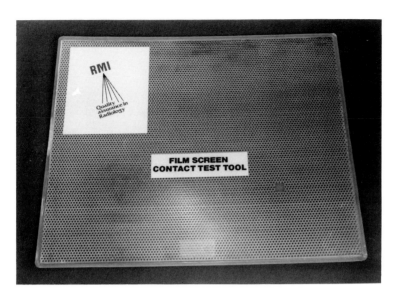

Causes of poor film–screen contact

(1) Badly mounted screens in the cassette
(2) Defects on the screen
(3) Damaged cassette
(4) Air trapped in the cassette

A test for contact between film and screen

A perforated sheet of metal is needed, 1 mm in thickness with holes of 2.5 mm diameter at intervals of 4 mm between the centre of the holes.[8] The sheet of metal should be large enough to cover the film and screen being used. This item of equipment, called a film–screen contact test tool (see Figure 2.10), can be purchased at a price of £92 (1985/6 price).

The cassette is loaded with film and the metal sheet or test tool placed over the cassette. The film is exposed at 50 kV with the appropriate intensity to give a density of 2 (see Chapter 3) and processed. The developed film should show a uniform density; darker areas mean a lack of contact between film and screen.

CARE AND HANDLING OF INTENSIFYING SCREENS

The screens should be inspected regularly to check there is no distortion or warping. They must be cleaned to remove any contamination such as dust. A record should be kept of when they are cleaned, and this information should also be noted on the outside of the cassette.

To clean the intensifying screens

Use a soft brush to remove any dust, and an antistatic cleaner, or a cleaner suggested by the manufacturer, and gently wipe in a circular fashion. A dry cloth is needed to remove surplus moisture. The cassette containing the screens is then placed in an upright position slightly opened, but not exposed to direct light, to allow the screens to dry completely. If the screens are left in a damp condition the surface may distort, and mould can form which will cause the phosphor layer to deteriorate.[9] If the screens are carefully handled they will last for years.

Cost of intensifying screens

This depends mainly on the size, type of screen and manufacturer.
   Calcium tungstate screens range from £15 to £60 per pair (1985/6 prices), with sizes from 18 × 24 cm to 35 × 43 cm.
   Rare earth screens range from £27 to £155 per pair (1985/6 prices), with sizes as above.

CASSETTES

The cassette is a light-tight container which protects the film. There are different varieties available depending on the type of film, or procedure, to be used.[10]

Cassettes containing duplitised screen-type film

These cassettes are unloaded and loaded with film in the darkroom under safe-light conditions unless a daylight system (see later in this chapter) is used, and then darkroom facilities are not needed.
   The cassette opens like a book and is hinged on one side (see Figure 2.11). The front of the cassette is deeper than the back and is called the 'well'. It contains the front intensifying screen and sometimes a portion for

Figure 2.11: Cassette containing intensifying screens. (Reproduced by permission of David Jenkins and MTP Press Ltd.)

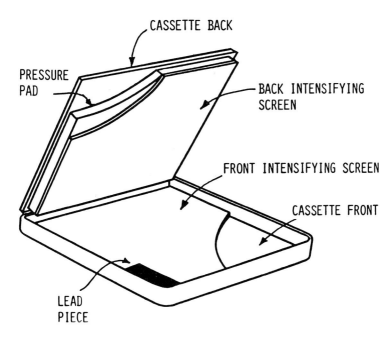

patient identification called the lead blocker. The 'well' of the cassette is made of plastic or a metal of low atomic number, such as aluminium. It is radiolucent and attenuates only a very small amount of radiation. Carbon fibre is now preferred, because even less of the primary beam is absorbed with a consequent reduction in dose to the patient (see Hufton *et al.*, in Further Reading list).

The back of the cassette used to be made from steel, but nowadays it is made of plastic to make the cassette lighter. It contains the back intensifying screen and the pressure pad, which is a plastic sponge, or felt material, which helps give good film-screen contact. Between the pressure pad and the back of the cassette is lead foil to absorb secondary radiation. The internal surfaces of the cassette are blackened to help prevent any external light getting into the cassette and fogging the sensitive film (see Chapter 4). The external surface has information regarding the type of screen mounted in the cassette.

Various clips are used to fasten the cassette, from sliding locking bars to metal springs of stainless steel. They all maintain pressure to keep the cassette light-tight and also to give good film-screen contact. Some cassettes are rigid and flat-backed and others slightly curved in construction but lay flat when closed. The curved type allows more expulsion of air

35

Figure 2.12: Curved non-rigid construction allows better film–screen contact. (Reproduced by permission of Kodak Ltd.)

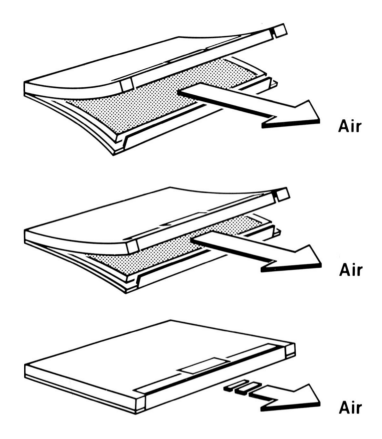

when the cassette is closed (see Figure 2.12) which the manufacturers suggest gives an even better film–screen contact.

The cassettes are usually supplied with intensifying screens already mounted, and depending on type and size required vary from £50 to £180 (1985/6 prices).

Daylight system

Screen-type film is automatically loaded and unloaded from a cassette in daylight conditions. There are two types of system for this process — the compact daylight system and the modular system (see Manufacturers' Literature).

The compact daylight system

This is a complete unit which will unload the film from the cassette in daylight, process the film and reload the cassette with film. The system is convenient as it includes magazines which carry the different sizes of film, and it gives advance warning when the films are running out. Some types of compact daylight systems give an automated read-out so the service engineer can check performance of the equipment. There are also safety and control devices to prevent incorrect operation. A disadvantage of the compact system is that if one part goes wrong the whole machine is out of action and therefore no films can be processed. It is an expensive unit ranging from £25,000 to £35,000 (1985/6 prices).

The modular system

This is made up of two separate units — a film dispenser which loads the cassette with film in daylight, and an automatic processor which unloads the film from the cassette in daylight and then processes the film. The film dispenser is usually situated on a wall, close to the processor, but separate ones are needed for different-size films. This is a disadvantage if a large range of film sizes is required. However, as the units are not integrated if one part goes wrong the whole system does not stop working. This system is also expensive; the processor with daylight unloader can cost around £8000 and each film dispenser £2500 (1985/6 prices).

The daylight cassette

This is similar to the ordinary screen-type cassette already mentioned, but with slight modifications which allow the cassette to be automatically unloaded and loaded with film in daylight conditions.

In Du Pont cassettes three of the sides are sealed and the fourth is opened when the cassette is unloaded and loaded with film. At the opposite end to the side which opens is a pin, which will verify whether a film is loaded. It is quite difficult to open this cassette manually. The intensifying screens in the cassette have an extra protective coat to help reduce friction, and they also have very minute elevations to help stop the film sticking to the screen during unloading. There is good film–screen contact because the front and back screens are pressed together by a spring mechanism. The spring separates slightly during loading and unloading of the film.[10]

Agfa Gevaert daylight cassettes are lightweight, made of synthetic material, and the corners are rounded and of rubber. To keep good film–screen contact there is a magnetic rubber layer on the rear surface in the cassette and a metal foil in the front surface. To show whether the cassette is loaded or unloaded there is a coloured dot on the outside of the cassette which is sunken when the cassette is empty, and cannot be felt when loaded with film. This cassette can be opened manually and used as an ordinary screen-type cassette.

The Kodak and 3M daylight cassettes are similar. They are both light-weight, durable and slightly curved to expel air for good film–screen contact. They can also be opened manually, and unloaded and loaded with film in the darkroom.

All these cassettes have small windows which allow an identification camera to be used for patient details (see below). Their screens will inevit-ably last longer, as there is minimal handling if automatically loaded and unloaded. Less dirt and dust is able to get to the intensifying screens so there will be fewer film faults (see Chapter 4).

The daylight cassettes are supplied with the intensifying screens and cost from £50 to £180 (1985/6 prices) depending on the size and type required.

Identification camera

Using the identification camera patient details can be recorded on the

Figure 2.13: Identification camera. (Courtesy of Agfa Gevaert.)

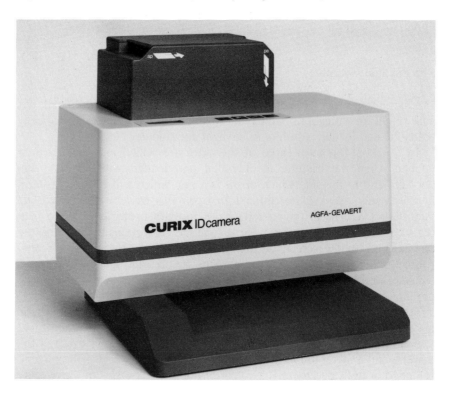

film.[10] The patient data is typed onto a card, in an area of approximately 8 × 3 cm, and inserted into the identification camera. After the imaging procedure the cassette is positioned into the camera so its identification window is in the correct place, or the machine will not function (see Figure 2.13). The machine slides back the cover on the identification window and the camera photographs the patient data onto the film. A signal is given when the exposure has been made. On some models, time and date can also be shown, because the camera has an internal clock. The information appears on the film as white letters on a black background. The time taken for this procedure is from 2 to 4 seconds, and it can be done in normal room lighting.

The identification cameras are reasonably small and compact. The dimensions of an Agfa Curix ID Camera are 39 cm in width, 33 cm in length and 34 cm in height, and the weight is approximately 10.5 kg. The price of this type of camera is £600. Some manufacturers produce identification cameras which can cost up to £1000 (1985/6 prices). They are expensive pieces of equipment but extremely useful. A cheaper method of patient identification on the film is by using an actinic marker, which costs from £145 (1985/6 prices).

Actinic markers

These are used for patient identification when the film is unloaded in the darkroom under safe-light conditions.[10] It is important that a lead blocker is used in the cassette so that a small part of the film has not been exposed to radiation or the actinic marking will not work.

The actinic marker can be recessed into the darkroom bench so it does not take up a great deal of space, as seen in Figure 2.14. The marker has a

Figure 2.14: Actinic marker recessed into bench top. (Reproduced by permission of David Jenkins and MTP Press Ltd.)

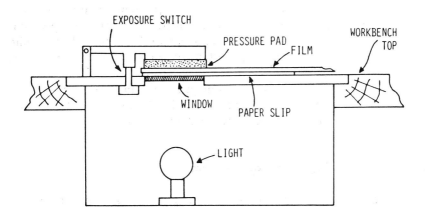

Figure 2.15: Film stops help correct positioning of the film. (Reproduced by permission of David Jenkins and MTP Press Ltd.)

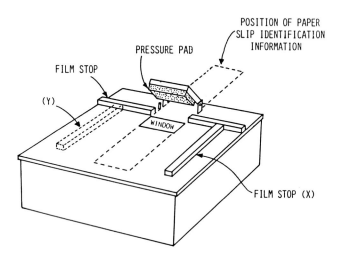

window approximately 2.5 cm in width and 7 cm in length with a small light bulb underneath. The box can be made of aluminium, and the whole marker weighs about 2.3 kg.

Patient details can either be typed or written, using a dark colour pen, onto a card. The area used on this card should not be larger than the window of the actinic marker. The card is then put into the marker. The film is positioned so that the area under the lead blocker is now under the window of the marker. The film stops, on the marker, help to correctly position the film (see Figure 2.15).

The pressure pad of the actinic marker is placed over the window, which will cause an exposure from the lamp. The time for the exposure will have been pre-set depending on whether a screen-type film or direct exposure film is used, and the lamp automatically switches off when the exposure is completed. The writing on the card is opaque to the light, and as the film and card are in contact, an image will appear on the film as white letters against a black background.

This method is very effective, but one problem is placing the wrong part of the film under the marker. If the area under the window of the marker has already been irradiated the marker will not be effective.

Cassettes containing direct exposure film

If the direct exposure film is not in a ready pack envelope (see Chapter 4),

40

it is necessary to place it in a light-tight holder in the darkroom under safe-light conditions.

A plastic envelope can be used which has a strengthened back with a lead foil lining to absorb scatter, and a radiolucent front with a matt black colour inside to help prevent fogging of the film from external light. The envelope is fastened with a Velcro fastener. It is important to ensure the envelope is light-tight as these envelopes are easily damaged and care must be taken with handling.

The direct exposure film which is in a 'ready pack' envelope does not require a cassette. However to give the film rigidity and sometimes better image quality it can be placed in a cardboard film holder. The cardboard holder has two pieces of cardboard hinged together with a lead foil lining to absorb scatter.

Kodak have produced a lightweight cassette for use with 'ready pack' film, which contains a copper screen as described earlier in this chapter. The cassette does not need to be carried to the darkroom because the film is in a 'ready pack' envelope, and only one cassette per treatment room is needed. However if screen-type film is used the cassette is unloaded in the darkroom and more cassettes may be required per treatment room.

Gridded cassette

This is a screen-type cassette plus a secondary radiation grid, usually parallel in construction (see later in this chapter). The grid is placed in the 'well' of the cassette in front of the intensifying screen (see Figure 2.16). The information about the type of grid used should be noted on the outside of the cassette. The gridded cassette can cost from £20 to £60 (1985/6 prices) plus the cost of the required grid (see later in this chapter).

Xeroradiographic cassette

There is no film in this cassette as the image produced is made on a charged plate (see Chapter 1). The cassette contains a thin layer of selenium on top of a thicker layer of aluminium and is known as the plate (see Figure 2.17). The plate is automatically loaded into the cassette after being charged in the conditioner (see Chapter 1). Excessive pressure must not be placed on the cassette, as this will cause a discharge on the plate, and the latent image will not be produced when the plate is irradiated. The cost of the cassette is £257 and the plate costs £185 (1985/6 prices).

Figure 2.16: Structure of gridded cassette. (Reproduced by permission of David Jenkins and MTP Press Ltd.)

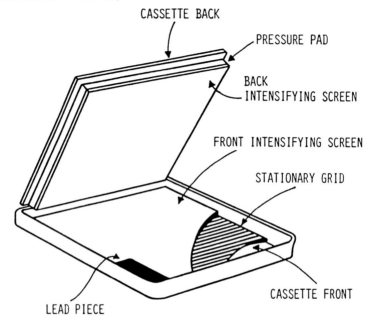

Figure 2.17: Xeroradiographic cassette. (Reproduced by permission of David Jenkins and MTP Press Ltd.)

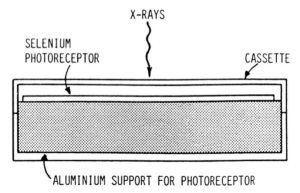

Cassette containing single-sided film

Single-sided film can be used for monitor photography when imaging directly from a cathode ray tube (see Chapter 7). The cassette used for this procedure is rather specialised. As well as enclosing the film in a light-tight casing it contains a slide which is pulled out so that the film can be exposed by the cathode ray tube (for more details see Manufacturers' Literature, Agfa Gevaert, Scopix Cassette).

HANDLING AND CARE OF CASSETTES

It is important to check cassettes regularly for any loose screws, hinges or locks, and to see that there is no obvious damage to the cassette. The cassettes will last for years if treated carefully.

A cassette should be carried between the body and the arm, and not just by the hand to avoid being dropped too often. If the cassette is going to be in contact with liquid a waterproof cover can be placed over it for protection. When the cassette is in contact with the patient, to help prevent cross-infection it should be cleaned with a disinfectant.

Mounting intensifying screens in a cassette

When buying a new screen-type cassette the intensifying screens are usually in place; however if old screens are being replaced, the new screens have to be mounted. It is important that the cassette to be used is not damaged in any way. If there is a lead blocker for identification purposes in the cassette the screen is carefully cut to avoid this.

A cassette used with duplitised film requires a front and back screen. The adhesive tapes are removed from the front screen and it is placed into the well of the cassette, phosphor surface uppermost. The back screen is placed on top of the front screen, with the phosphor surface towards the front screen. The adhesive tapes are removed from the back screen and the cassette is closed. After a short period of time the screens should be examined to see if they are correctly in place.[9]

SECONDARY RADIATION GRIDS

Secondary or scattered radiation is one of the major causes of poor-quality images. This scattered radiation depends on the subject which is imaged, the total area of the image and the energy of the primary radiation (see Chapter 3).

To try to reduce scatter reaching the film emulsion and degrading the image the area in question should be limited to a minimum by closing down the collimators or light beam diaphragm (see Chapter 5), and using a lower kilovoltage which gives less scatter in the forward direction. To help lessen the problem even more a secondary radiation grid or scatter grid can be used. The grid should allow the primary beam of radiation to produce the image and absorb as much of the secondary radiation as possible, but in practice some of the primary radiation is absorbed as well as the scatter.

Construction of a secondary radiation grid

The grid is made up of long thin strips of lead which are known as lines. This is called the grid lattice and can vary from 20 to 60 lines per cm. There is radiolucent material in between the lead strips, usually of aluminium or plastic. (Carbon fibre is now preferred; see Hufton *et al.*, Further Reading.) The grid is sealed in a durable radiolucent material, and coated with lacquer so that moisture cannot get in and damage the structure. There are different size grids made for the different sizes of film and cassette combinations.[11]

Grid ratio

The ratio of the height of the lead strips to the distance between them is the grid ratio (see Figure 2.18). The higher the ratio the more secondary radiation is absorbed, which will give a better-quality image, but more incident radiation is needed if the same density (see Chapter 3) is required for the image.

Figure 2.18: Grid ratio. (Reproduced by permission of Wardray Products (Clerkenwell) Ltd.)

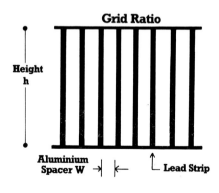

Grid Ratio $= \dfrac{h}{w}$ h = height   W = width of spaces

For example, height is 1.6 mm
width of spaces 0.2 mm
Grid Ratio is 8:1

Grid factor (GF)

The exposure needs to be increased to compensate for the loss of primary and scattered radiation when using a grid. The amount of increase is shown by the grid factor,[12] and the factor varies between two and six. A definition for the grid factor is shown below:

$$GF = \frac{\text{Exposure required with a grid}}{\text{Exposure required without a grid}}$$

to produce the same density on the image in each case.

Types of secondary radiation grids

There are two kinds of grid — parallel and focused — and these can be made either in a linear or a crossed fashion.

The linear arrangement has the length of its lead strips all in the same direction. The crossed type is usually two linear-type grids, one on top of the other with their lead strips crossing at right angles.

The linear pattern grid is generally used in preference to the crossed type because, although the crossed type grid will remove more scattered radiation, at least double the amount of exposure is required for a similar density image. Another problem of the crossed type is that the lead strips are more noticeable when the image is viewed than with the equivalent linear arrangement.

Parallel grids

All the lead strips are parallel to each other over the whole area of the grid. A disadvantage of the parallel grid is the loss of primary radiation which is absorbed by the lead strips because of the spreading of the beam, and which will produce an inferior image (see Figure 2.19). It means that there is not uniform density over the whole area of the beam unless the field size is below about 10 × 10 cm. Loss of primary radiation can also be caused if the grid is not placed perpendicular to the radiation beam.

Focused grids

The disadvantage of loss of primary radiation with a parallel grid is overcome with a focused grid. The lead strips are angled more towards the edge, as the beam spreads out, and at the centre of the beam they are

Figure 2.19: Parallel grid. (Reproduced by permission of Wardray Products (Clerkenwell) Ltd.)

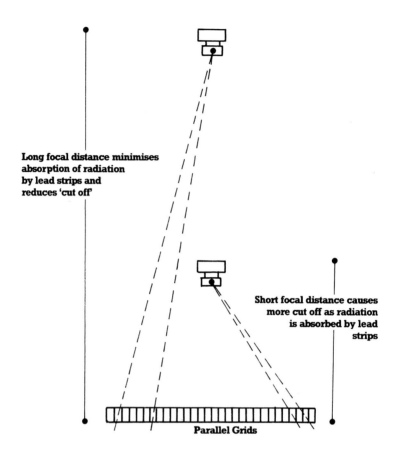

Long focal distance minimises
absorption of radiation
by lead strips and
reduces 'cut off'

Short focal distance causes
more cut off as radiation
is absorbed by lead
strips

Parallel Grids

parallel to the central axis (see Figure 2.20). This grid can only be used at a specified distance and correctly centred, otherwise the gain in uniform density across the beam is lost. The focused grid must also be used perpendicular to the beam of radiation and with the correct side towards the source of radiation.

Cost of grids

Depending on the type and size required a secondary radiation grid can cost from about £200 to £900 (1985/6 prices).

Figure 2.20: Focused grid. (Reproduced by permission of Wardray Products (Clerkenwell) Ltd.)

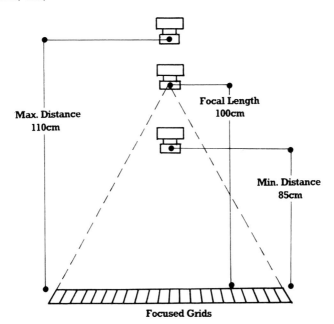

Focused Grids

Use of secondary radiation grids in radiotherapy

For localisation of the treatment field it is useful to use a secondary radiation grid when trying to image large areas, especially in the abdomen and pelvis, as a great deal of scatter is produced. Other areas where a grid may be helpful to produce a better image are where there is dense bone, such as the skull and spine, and especially if the spine is being imaged with the patient prone and the film underneath the patient. When high kV (above 80 kV) is used for a localising procedure (see Chapter 6) a grid will help reduce secondary radiation.

REFERENCES

1. Kodak, 'X-ray recording materials', *Fundamentals of Radiographic Photography*, vol. II, pp. 11–13.
2. Meredith, W.J. and Massey, J.B. (1977) *Fundamental Physics of Radiology*, 3rd edn, Wright, Bristol, pp. 85–93.
3. Wilks, R. (1982) *Principles of Radiological Physics*, Churchill Livingstone, Edinburgh, pp. 368–71.

4. Eastman Kodak (1976) *Screen Imaging*, Image Insight 3, Eastman Kodak Company.
5. 3M (1985) *Rare Earth Systems*, 3M Diagnostic Imaging Markets.
6. Jenkins, D. (1980) *Radiographic Photography and Imaging Processes*, MTP Press, Lancaster, pp. 38–9.
7. Plane, J.H. (1985) 'Comparison of radiographic technique', *Radiography*, vol. 51, no. 598, pp. 211–14.
8. Kodak, *Fundamentals of Radiographic Photography*, vol. II. pp. 21–4.
9. Chesney, D.N. and Chesney, M.O. (1981) *Radiographic Imaging*, 4th edn, Blackwell Scientific Publications, Oxford, pp. 113, 117–21.
10. Jenkins, D. (1980) *Radiographic Photography and Imaging Processes*, MTP Press, Lancaster, pp. 78–83, 241–2, 158–61.
11. Liebel–Flarshem (1983) *Characteristics and Applications of X-ray Grids*, Liebel–Flarshem Company, Sybron.
12. Gifford, D. (1984) *A Handbook of Physics for Radiologists and Radiographers*, John Wiley and Sons, Chichester, pp. 281–8.

Private communications

M. Clark; T. Cropper (Marketing Education Centre, Kodak); N. Smith (Agfa Gevaert); J. Stock.

Manufacturers' literature

Agfa Gevaert, Diagnostic Imaging Systems Medical Division Price List, 1985.
Agfa Gevaert Curix MR4 Film/Screen System.
Agfa Gevaert Curix ID Camera.
Agfa Gevaert Scopix Cassette.
Du Pont, Superior technology for a better diagnosis, Cronex Quanta System (Screens/Film system).
Du Pont, Compact Daylight System.
Du Pont, Modular Daylight System.
Kodak, Medical Buyers Guide to the DHSS, 1985.
Kodak, X-Omatic Intensifying Screens and X-Omat Films.
Kodak, 'Lanex' Intensifying Screens and Ortho Films.
3M, Diagnostic Imaging Systems Product Directory. Wardray Products, Clerkenwell Ltd., Price List, 1985.

FURTHER READING

Chesney, D.N. and Chesney, M.O. (1981) *Radiographic Imaging*, 4th edn, Blackwell Scientific Publications, Oxford, pp. 90–7.
Hufton, A., Crosthwaite, C.M., Davies, J.M. and Robinson, L.A. (1987) 'Low attenuation material for table tops cassettes and grids: a review', *Radiography*, vol. 53, no. 607, pp. 17–18.
Meredith, W.J. and Massey, J.B. (1977) *Fundamental Physics of Radiology*, 3rd edn, Wright, Bristol, pp. 191–205.

3

Image Quality and Sensitometry

IMAGE QUALITY

The image produced should show good definition, which means it has a sharp outline with fine detail. Unsharpness, contrast and noise will affect the definition of the image.

Sharpness

A distinct boundary which is shown between structures means the image is sharp. It can be described as subjective and objective sharpness.

Subjective sharpness

The interpretation by the viewer will give a personal opinion of the sharpness of the image. It also depends on the quality of the viewing equipment used.[1]

Objective sharpness

The sharpness of the image can be measured; it is the width of the edge of blurring or unsharpness between adjacent structures.

Some of the causes of unsharpness or blurring of an image

Geometric

X-rays are produced when electrons are accelerated from a cathode to a metal anode, which acts as a target, in an X-ray tube. The area where the electrons hit the target is called the focal spot. Depending on the size of the focal spot a penumbra is formed which causes geometric unsharpness on the image (see Figure 3.1). An ideal focal spot would be a very small point, but in practice it has a certain size and is sometimes called a line focus.

Figure 3.1: Diagram showing the larger the focus the greater the penumbra. (Reproduced by permission of Kodak Ltd.)

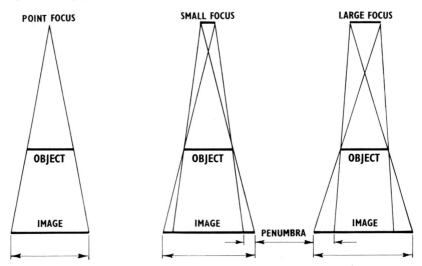

Effective focal spot

The actual or real focal spot is where the electrons hit the anode, but the projection of this area at right angles is called the effective or apparent focal spot. The size of the effective focal spot depends on the angle of the anode which can be from 8° to 22° in an X-ray tube. The smaller the angle of the anode the smaller is the effective focal spot (see Figure 3.2). The size of the focal spot as quoted by manufacturers usually refers to the effective focal spot and can be from 0.2 × 0.2 mm to 2 × 2 mm. A small focal spot will give the image greater sharpness than a large focal spot.[2] (For more details on focal spot and anode angle see Chapter 5.)

Penumbra

This is a partial shadow cast when radiation is emitted from a finite area rather than a point. It will cause a certain degree of unsharpness of the image, and will depend on the size of the effective focal spot, the distance from the actual focal spot to the object and the distance between the film and the object being imaged (see Figure 3.3). A small penumbra and greater image clarity require:

> Small focal spot
> Large distance between object and focal spot
> Small distance between object and film

The size of the penumbra can be measured using the information in Figure 3.4.

Figure 3.2: Diagram showing different sizes of effective focal spot. (Reproduced by permission of Kodak Ltd.)

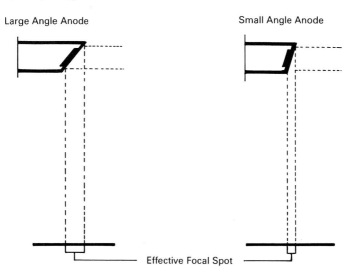

Large Angle Anode

Small Angle Anode

Effective Focal Spot

Figure 3.3: Larger penumbra for 2 than for 1. Object further from film for 2. Smaller penumbra for 3 than for 2. Long focus to film distance for 3. (Reproduced by permission of Kodak Ltd.)

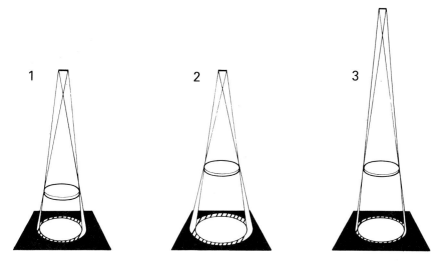

1

2

3

Movement

The movement of either the patient (and this usually refers to involuntary movement), film or X-ray tube will cause unsharpness of the image. It

51

Figure 3.4: Measurement of penumbra. (Reproduced by permission of Kodak Ltd.)
p = penumbra (u.v.)
f = effective focus (xy)
i = object to film distance
o = focus to object distance.
By using the geometry of the triangles xyz and uvz

$$\frac{p}{i} = \frac{f}{o}; \text{ therefore } p = \frac{f \times i}{o}.$$

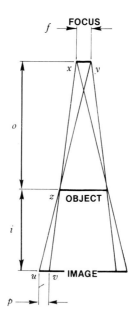

depends on the rate of movement, by how much, for how long and to a lesser degree in which direction.[1]

An acceptable amount of involuntary movement is 0.1 mm for good image quality. When imaging a patient in the chest region it has been calculated that movement caused by the heart beating is approximately 3 mm per second. Therefore to achieve a sharp image using 0.1 mm as a tolerance level, the exposure time should not be greater than 0.03 second.

Photographic

Intensifying screens

These are used with X-ray film and, when irradiated, light photons are emitted from the screens and produce a latent image in the X-ray film emulsion (see Chapter 4). The following characteristics of the screens cause unsharpness of the image: the emission of light in many directions, causing the light to spread out slightly before it reaches the emulsion of the film; lack of close contact between film and screens in the cassette, accentuating this spreading of the beam; and the use of two intensifying screens, which creates the cross-over effect. (For details of these effects see Chapter 2.)

Duplitised film

This has two emulsions (see Chapter 1) and shows a certain amount of unsharpness caused by the parallax effect.[1] Two images are formed, one in each emulsion, and if the film is viewed at the same angle as the radiation strikes the emulsions the image will be superimposed. However, films are generally viewed at right angles, and not all the radiation strikes the film at 90° so a slight unsharpness of the image may be seen (see Figure 3.5). This is more obvious when the films are viewed when 'wet' — for instance if a manual processor is used (see Chapter 4) — but not so noticeable when the films are processed in the automatic processor (see Chapter 4) and are viewed when 'dry'.

Figure 3.5: Parallax effect. (Reproduced by permission of Kodak Ltd.)

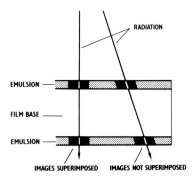

Summary of the causes of unsharpness

Geometric Ug
Movement Um
Photographic Up

(For further information see Reference 1.)

Total unsharpness can be calculated using the following formula:

$$U \text{ Total} = \sqrt[3]{Ug^3 + Um^3 + Up^3}$$

If no movement is involved the calculation would follow the formula:

$$U \text{ Total} = \sqrt{Ug^2 + Up^2}$$

CONTRAST

There are several different terms which relate to the contrast of an image.[3,4]

Objective contrast

The difference in the degree of blackening or density between two areas of the image is called objective contrast. It is measured by using a densito-meter (see later in this chapter).

Subjective contrast

The subjective contrast is the viewer's own opinion of the difference in density between two areas of the image.

Subject contrast

Subject contrast is formed because of the different attenuation of the radiation, by the subject, when being imaged. It depends on the physical density or thickness, the atomic number of the various parts of the subject and also on the energy of the radiation being used to produce the image.[5]

The main attenuation process that concerns the production of an image for localisation purposes (see Chapter 6) is photoelectric absorption. At low energies, such as 50 kV, photoelectric absorption is proportional to the cube of the atomic number of the material being exposed and inversely proportional to the cube of the energy. This means substances with a high atomic number irradiated at low energies will greatly attenuate the radiation beam.[6]

When considering images produced for verification using the radiotherapy treatment units, above 0.5 MeV, the Compton scatter attenuation process becomes more important. The atomic number of the material is less relevant, but it is the electron density of the material that is the guide to the amount of attenuation of the beam; the greater the electron density the more attenuation occurs.

At even higher energies, above 1.02 MeV, the pair production process takes place, and it is proportional to the atomic number, so the higher the atomic number of the material the more the beam is attenuated. Unlike the other processes attenuation of the beam by pair production increases with higher energies. In practice pair production is not really important until about 10 MeV, and with materials of very high atomic number.

The difference in density (see later in this chapter) of the image is caused by the subject contrast. For instance an exposure at 60 kV bone, which has a higher atomic number (13.8) than soft tissue (7.2) and fat (5.92), will attenuate the radiation more due to the photoelectric effect, and will allow less radiation to reach the emulsion of the film. This area seen on the viewed image will be less dense, and will show as different shades of light grey. The soft tissue and fat will attenuate the radiation less, and cause more radiation to get to the emulsion of the film and show as darker areas on the image. The thickness of the area being imaged is also important; a thicker part of bone such as the head or femur will attenuate the radiation more and show less density on the image than a thinner part of bone such as the scapula.

At higher energies, when the radiotherapy treatment units are used for verification, Compton scatter is the main process of attenuation, and as the parts of the subject imaged have similar electron densities (bone 3.0×10^{23}, soft tissue 3.36×10^{23}, and fat 3.34×10^{23}), they all attenuate the radiation in a similar fashion. This will cause the subject contrast to be low, and there will not be a great difference in density on the film, so it will be difficult to distinguish the different structures on the image. Another problem at these energies is the great amounts of scatter produced in a forward direction, which will give an overall fogging or greyness to the film. This can be partially overcome by using lead or copper screens with the film (see Chapter 2).

Radiographic contrast

Radiographic contrast is the variations in density made on the image, because of the different attenuation of radiation through the subject. From the above explanation on subject contrast, it can be seen that at low energies the radiographic contrast is high, but at the higher energies used for verification on the radiotherapy treatment units, the radiographic contrast is low.

For localisation purposes, if the energy of the radiation needs to be increased (e.g. 100 kV) to penetrate the area being imaged, this produces more scattered radiation in a forward direction and will reduce radiographic contrast. Therefore for better contrast of the image it will help to keep the area of radiation as small as possible, and to use a secondary radiation grid (see Chapter 2). Unfortunately, by using this grid it is necessary to increase the intensity of the radiation through the subject to get an acceptable image.

Film contrast

The film contrast is the amount of contrast the film is able to show. It is a property of the film emulsion and depends on the range of grain sizes in the emulsion (see Chapter 1). It can be measured from the average gradient of the characteristic curve (see later in this chapter).

NOISE

Noise consists of artefacts, film grain and mottle, and it makes the image more difficult to interpret accurately.[7,8]

Artefacts

These are marks or scratches on an image, and can be caused by processing, bad handling, or incorrect storage. The most common cause is dirty or damaged screens (see Chapter 4).

Film grain

When primary radiation is scattered in the emulsion of the film electrons are produced, and if the electrons are moving very slowly they can give up all their energy in one area to the halide crystals. This area then becomes developable (see Chapter 4), which will give a grainy appearance to the image. Film grain is negligible compared with the mottle caused when using intensifying screens.

Mottle

This is made up of structure mottle and quantum mottle.

Structure mottle

This occurs because of differences in the structure of the intensifying screen. For instance, clumping of the phosphor crystals will cause a slight density variation, which is not due to the radiographic exposure. However, like film grain this is a small problem compared with quantum mottle.

Quantum mottle

This gives the image a mottled appearance because the radiation is being absorbed randomly by the intensifying screen and exposes the film emulsion unevenly. It is more noticeable when using a high-speed film–screen combination (see Chapter 2).

In theory a simplistic view is the raindrop analogy. When it just starts to rain the raindrops can be seen on the pavement; however with a great downfall of rain the whole pavement becomes wet and so the separate rain-drops are not noticed. To liken this to quantum mottle, when a fast film–screen combination is used a small amount of radiation is needed to expose the film, and quantum mottle is more visible on the image. For the same density image, and using a slower film–screen combination, more radiation is needed to expose the film and quantum mottle is less visible.

It is therefore important to strike a balance and have a film–screen combination which produces least exposure to the patient, and optimum detail needed for the image.

SENSITOMETRY

Sensitometry is a quantitative evaluation of how a film emulsion responds to radiation and chemical processing (see Chapter 4). It is shown by

Figure 3.6: Characteristic curve. (Reproduced by permission of Kodak Ltd.)

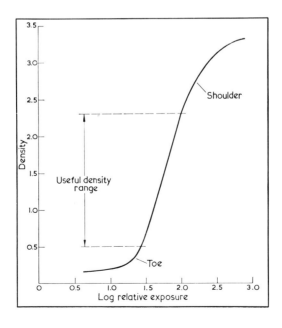

producing a characteristic curve (see later in this chapter) on a graph, plotting density against logarithm relative exposure (see Figure 3.6). It is used to compare films, screens and film–screen combinations as well as being used for monitoring the efficiency of the processor. The details of processor monitoring using sensitometry are in Chapter 4.

Exposure

With reference to sensitometry the exposure is the amount of radiation reaching the film.

$$\text{Exposure} = \text{Intensity} \times \text{Time } (E = I \times t)$$

There are other interpretations of the word exposure; for instance the radiographic conditions such as kV, mA, and time can be called the exposure (see Chapters 5 and 6). The amount of radiation a patient receives is also sometimes referred to as exposure.

Logarithm relative exposure (log rel E)

This expression is used when plotting the characteristic curve. The logarithm scale enables a small number scale to be used to represent a large range of relative exposure values.

Relative exposure

The exposures used increase at the same rate; for instance they are doubled

Figure 3.7: Density $= \log^{10} \dfrac{\text{Ii}}{\text{It}}$ (Reproduced by permission of Kodak Ltd.)

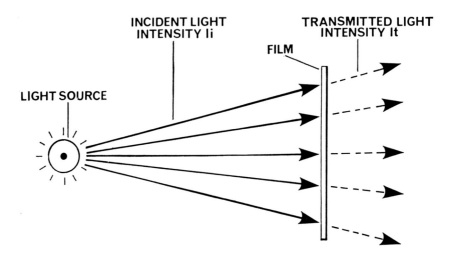

INCIDENT LIGHT
INTENSITY Ii

TRANSMITTED LIGHT
INTENSITY It

FILM

LIGHT SOURCE

each time, and are given using the same equipment to produce the image and in this way relate to each other.

Density

The amount of blackening on a film can be measured using a densitometer, and is called density. It is the logarithm of the ratio of the light incident on the film to the light transmitted by the film (see Figure 3.7).

Densitometer

When a small area of the film is illuminated, the light transmitted by that part of the film is detected by a photocell in the densitometer. A read-out of the density can then be seen on a meter with a scale, or in a digital form.

PRODUCING A CHARACTERISTIC CURVE

Time scale sensitometry

One method of producing a characteristic curve is by time scale sensitometry.[9] An X-ray unit is used to give an X-ray film a series of exposures, for

Figure 3.8: Using time scale sensitometry to produce a characteristic curve. In this diagram two films are being compared. (Reproduced by permission of David Jenkins and MTP Press Ltd.)

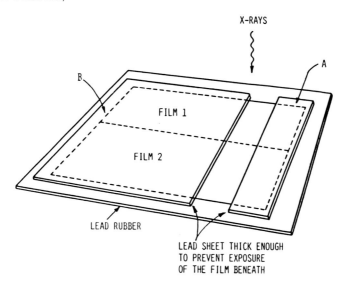

example, 2 mAs, 4 mAs, 8 mAs, 16 mAs, 32 mAs, etc. The kV and mA should not be changed — only the time.

The film is covered with lead rubber, gradually uncovering sections for increasing exposure (see Figure 3.8). A large distance between the focal spot and film should be used, at least 1.5 m, and a small beam size to avoid variation in intensity across the area being irradiated. A copper filter (0.6 mm thick) is placed in the path of the radiation beam to approximate the attenuation of the patient, or the intensity of the radiation would completely darken the film. The beam of radiation should be centred on each section as it is exposed. A portion of the film can be covered all the time to measure the gross fog level (see later in this chapter). The film is then processed using standard conditions (see Chapter 4) and a densito-meter measures the different densities of the sections on the image. The densities are plotted on graph paper against the exposure which are turned into log values (for each doubling of the exposure the log value increases by 0.3).

Intensity scale sensitometry

Another way of producing a characteristic curve is by intensity scale

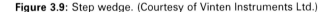

Figure 3.9: Step wedge. (Courtesy of Vinten Instruments Ltd.)

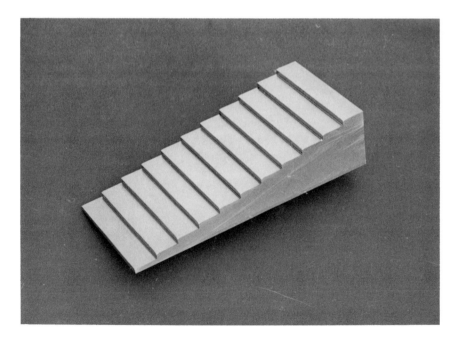

sensitometry.[9] A calibrated step wedge is used, which is of different thicknesses of a metal such as aluminium or copper (see Figure 3.9). The step wedge produces an equal amount of difference in intensities between each step, so that it is possible to plot the density against the step number. Only one exposure is needed from the X-ray set. The quality of the radiation reaching the film will change with the different thicknesses of metal in the step wedge. This method does not accurately show the characteristics of the film; however, the variation only accounts for a small discrepancy.

The easiest way of producing the image for a characteristic curve to be plotted is by using a light sensitometer,[9] and by not using an X-ray set at all.

Light sensitometer

Inside the sensitometer is a tungsten light with a green or blue filter depending on whether monochromatic or orthochromatic film is being used (see Chapter 1). A density step tablet divided into steps is incorporated in the sensitometer which allows a constant increasing fraction of light to be transmitted. On exposure by the light the step tablet is imaged onto the film (see Figure 3.10). If duplitised film is used both sides must be exposed under the sensitometer, unless the sensitometer automatically exposes both sides at the same time.

The film is processed using standard conditions, and the different densities of the various sections are measured using a densitometer and a characteristic curve plotted (see Figure 3.11).

THE CHARACTERISTIC CURVE[9]

Threshold value

This is the point where the film has started to respond to the radiographic exposure, and is shown at B on the characteristic curve in Figure 3.12.

Toe of the curve

This is the part of the characteristic curve from B to C in Figure 3.12 where the densities can vary from 0.1 to 0.5.

Straight-line portion

This is the part from C to D in Figure 3.12, and shows a steady increase in density from 0.5 to 2.5. It is sometimes difficult to distinguish the straight line portion as it tends to be more curved for some types of X-ray film, especially direct exposure film (see Figure 3.13).

Gross fog

An X-ray film will have a certain amount of density which is not from the radiographic exposure. It is caused by many things, for instance, film base (see Chapter 1); it also depends on handling, storage, processing and background radiation (see Chapter 4). The gross fog, which is sometimes referred to as base plus fog, basic fog or fog density, has a density usually from 0.15 to 0.25, and is shown in Figure 3.12 from A to B.

Figure 3.10: Step tablet produced from light sensitometer. (Courtesy of Agfa Gevaert.)

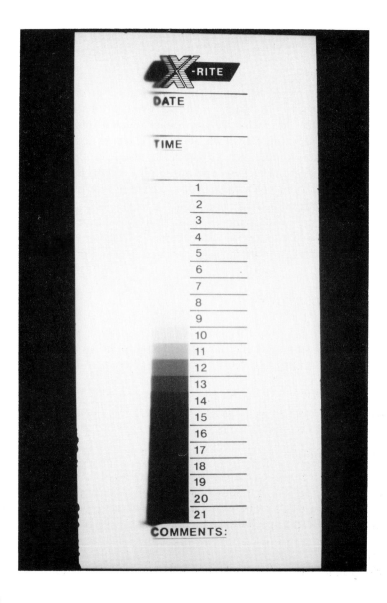

Net density

From the radiographic exposure which is used to produce the image, and after processing of the film, there is a net density. To find the net density, the gross fog is subtracted from the measured density of the image.

Figure 3.11: Characteristic curve produced using step tablet. (Courtesy of Agfa Gevaert.)

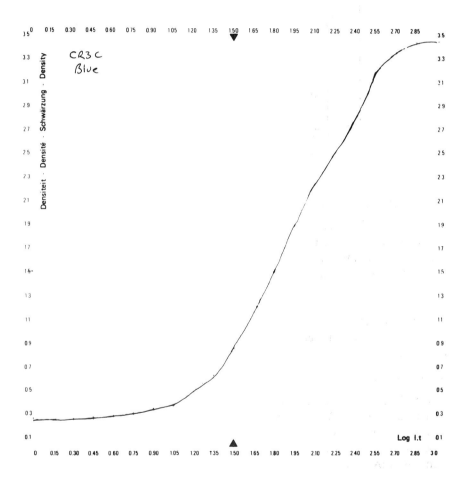

Figure 3.12: Characteristic curve. (Reproduced by permission of Kodak Ltd.)

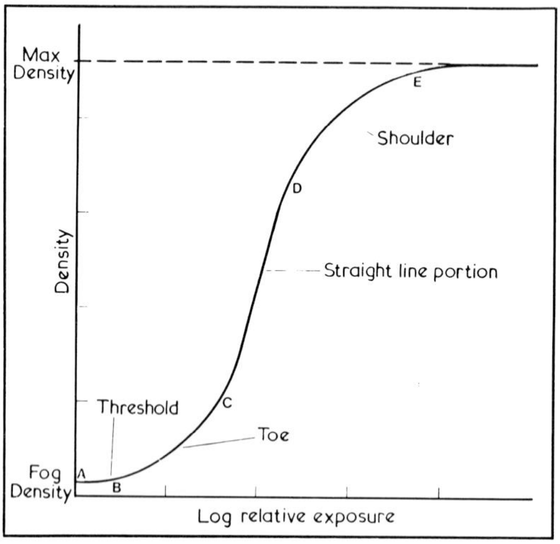

The useful density range

This is from 0.25 plus gross fog to 2.0 plus gross fog (see Figure 3.6). It is useful because it is the upper and lower range of density which the eye can perceive on the image. Above or below this range it is difficult for the eye to differentiate between the densities.

Shoulder

The shoulder is from D to E in Figure 3.12 and there is not much difference in density for an increase in exposure. The shoulder gradually reaches maximum density.

Maximum density

When all the silver halide crystals have been developed in an area of the film (see Chapter 4), this point is called maximum density, and shown above E in Figure 3.12. It is sometimes referred to as D max. For screen type film the density is between 3.2 and 4.0, and for direct exposure film it is above 6.0.

Solarisation or recombination

When the exposure increases above maximum density the density on the film then starts to decrease. This happens because the silver formed begins to break down (see Chapter 4). The process is called solarisation or recombination, and a tremendous amount of radiation is needed before it

Figure 3.13: Film K, screen–type film exposed using intensifying screens; Film L, screen–type film exposed to direct X-rays; Film M, direct exposure film exposed to direct X-rays. (Reproduced by permission of Kodak Ltd.)

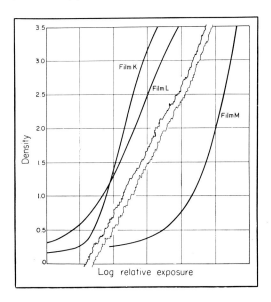

starts to happen. Manufacturers put this effect to use for making copy film.

Copy film

This is solarised by the manufacturer and acts in the opposite manner to an ordinary X-ray film when exposed to light. Copy film is single-sided film, and the emulsion is placed towards the emulsion of the film to be copied, which is exposed to ultraviolet or white light.

For an area of high density on the plain X-ray film only a small amount of light passes through to expose the copy film, which will show as a high-density area on the copy film. The low-density areas on the ordinary X-ray film will transmit more light and cause less density on the copy film. In this way an exact replica can be made of the original film.

Use of the characteristic curve

The following information shows how the characteristic curve can be used to find the average gradient (contrast), latitude and speed of an X-ray film. Comparisons can then be made with different types of film, different screens and different film–screen combinations to find the most useful and efficient imaging system for the procedure in question.

Figure 3.14: Measurement of average gradient.

D_2 = density at point A
D_1 = density at point B
$\log E_2$ = log rel. exposure at
        point A
$\log E_1$ = log rel. exposure at
        point B

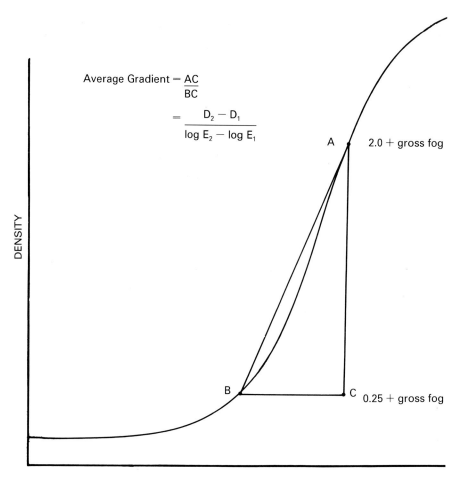

Average Gradient $= \dfrac{AC}{BC}$

$$= \dfrac{D_2 - D_1}{\log E_2 - \log E_1}$$

A   2.0 + gross fog

B

C   0.25 + gross fog

DENSITY

LOG REL. EXPOSURE

Average gradient

The average gradient shows the contrast properties of a film emulsion. It is measured using the useful density range 0.25 plus gross fog and density 2.00 plus gross fog, and is the tangent of the angle formed between a line joining these two points and the relative exposure axis of the characteristic curve (see Figure 3.14). The steeper the slope of the characteristic curve the higher the contrast the film is able to show.

Latitude

Film latitude

The latitude of the film (see Figure 3.15) means the ability of the film to be able to respond to a range of exposures. If a film has a wide latitude, variation in exposures can be given and produce an acceptable image, but with a small latitude such a variation would make the film under- or over-exposed.

The latitude depends on the average gradient; if this increases the film latitude decreases. As contrast is measured using average gradient, latitude and contrast are reciprocal quantities.

Figure 3.15: Film B has wider latitude than Film A. (Reproduced by permission of Kodak Ltd.)

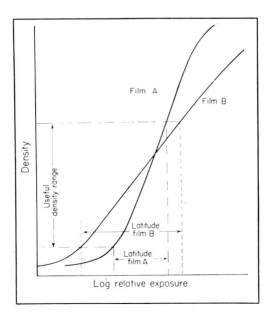

High contrast — small latitude
Low contrast — wide latitude

Exposure latitude

This is the range of exposures which can be given to the film and still produce a reasonable image. It will vary according to the subject being imaged, because of the different attenuation of the radiation through the subject.

Speed

The speed of a film shows how it responds to radiation. The more exposure needed to produce a given density, the slower the film. If the characteristic curve is closer to the density axis, the film will be faster (see Figure 3.16).

The film speed is measured at a certain level, the speed point, which is an international standard, so that different films can be compared. The speed point is measured at density 1.0 plus gross fog.

Figure 3.16: Diagram showing Film F is faster than Film G. (Reproduced by permission of Kodak Ltd.)

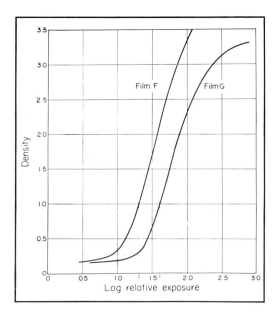

REFERENCES

1. Kodak, 'Radiographic quality', *Fundamentals of Radiographic Photography*, vol. III, pp. 11-22.
2. Kodak, 'Geometry of image formation', *Image Insight*, 2, pp. 2-12.
3. Kodak, 'Radiographic quality', *Fundamentals*, vol. III, pp. 3–6.
4. Kodak, 'Image quality control', *Fundamentals*, vol. I, pp. 7–9.
5. Kodak, 'X-ray recording materials, *Fundamentals*, vol. II, pp. 25–9.
6. Wilks, R. (1981) *Principles of Radiological Physics*, Churchill Livingstone, Edinburgh, pp. 395–430.
7. Kodak, 'Radiographic noise', *Image Insight*, 4, pp. 1–13, 17–19.
8. Fuji, 'Image quality in radiography', *Fuji Film Technical Handbook*, Fuji Photo Film Co., Ltd., Japan, p. 16.
9. Kodak, 'Image quality control', *Fundamentals*, vol. I, pp. 3–25.

Private communications

O. Deaville; P. Lowes.

FURTHER READING

Fuji, 'Fundamentals of sensitized materials', *Fuji Film Technical Handbook*, Fuji Photo Film Co., Ltd.
Fuji, 'Image quality in radiography', *Fuji Film Technical Handbook*, Fuji Photo

4

The Latent Image and Processing

When ionising radiation passes through a subject and on to an X-ray film a pattern is produced in the sensitive emulsion layer of the film. This is called the latent image.[1] This image cannot be seen by the eye until the film has been processed.

FORMATION OF THE LATENT IMAGE

There are many theories on the formation of the latent image, and the following is a brief simplified version of events.

Electron traps

The emulsion of an X-ray film consists of silver bromide crystals suspended in gelatin (see Chapter 1). Sulphur impurities contained in the gelatin, and physical defects in the silver bromide crystals, produce areas of low energy called electron traps which help form the latent image.

Bromine barrier

There is a bromine barrier around the silver bromide crystals because an excess of potassium bromide is used in the manufacture of the crystals. The excess of bromine ions which collect at the surface is balanced by mobile silver ions in the crystals, and this means that the crystals are electrically neutral.

Mobile silver ions

These help form the sensitivity centres, and the more stable development centres.

Sensitivity centres

High-energy electrons are produced when radiation is absorbed by the silver bromide crystals. Some of these high-energy electrons fall into the electron traps, and form sensitivity centres which are negatively charged.

Development centres

A sensitivity centre will attract a positive mobile silver ion which will combine with a free electron, produced by the attenuation of the incident radiation in the crystal, and form a silver atom. To make the sensitivity centre stable more high-energy electrons deposit at the centre and attract silver ions and free electrons to form atoms of silver. The centre will grow and eventually destroy the bromine barrier and break the surface of the crystal. It is now susceptible to development by specialised chemicals and is called a development centre.

These changes mainly occur in the crystals which have been exposed to radiation, and therefore there is a difference between the crystals which have received radiation and those which have not. When radiation is absorbed by the silver bromide crystals some of the bromine ions are converted into bromine atoms and are taken up by the gelatin. In this way the gelatin protects the latent image by preventing recombination of the bromine with the silver atoms.[2,3]

DEVELOPMENT OF THE LATENT IMAGE

The chemicals used in the developer solution are selective, and cause the exposed crystals with development centres to be converted into black metallic silver. The effect of the developer on the unexposed crystals is minimal.

Exposed silver bromide crystal

A break is made in the bromine barrier because of the development centres, and this allows the developer to penetrate. The crystal is reduced to black metallic silver because of the donation of electrons from the developer (see Figure 4.1). The bromine ions which are left go into the developer solution.

Unexposed silver bromide crystal

The bromine barrier is not broken and repels the electrons being donated by the developer (see Figure 4.1).

Fog

The unexposed crystals can be made developable by bad handling such as pressure on the film. This can also happen if the X-ray films are stored in an area of high temperature, with chemical fumes, or accidentally exposed to light or ionising radiation. This will cause blackening or density (see Chapter 3) on the film which is not due to the radiographic exposure (see Chapter 6) needed for the image, and is called fog.

Figure 4.1: Effect of bromine barrier. (Courtesy of Agfa Gevaert.)

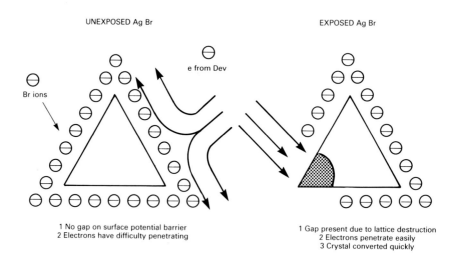

UNEXPOSED Ag Br

EXPOSED Ag Br

e from Dev

Br ions

1 No gap on surface potential barrier
2 Electrons have difficulty penetrating

1 Gap present due to lattice destruction
2 Electrons penetrate easily
3 Crystal converted quickly

Fixing

It is necessary to fix the developed image, otherwise the unexposed crystals will eventually turn to silver in daylight conditions. Fixing is also important for archiving purposes, so that films can be kept as a record. During fixing further development is prevented, the unexposed crystals are removed and at the same time the film is hardened to protect the emulsion from damage during handling.

Washing and drying

The film is washed to remove all excess chemicals and to prevent any further reactions. It is then dried so that it can be handled and viewed more easily.

COMPOSITION OF DEVELOPER FOR AUTOMATIC PROCESSORS[4,5]

Developing agents

These are in a concentrated liquid form and prepared for use by diluting with water. The chemicals used are phenidone and hydroquinone (PQ developers). They reduce the exposed silver bromide crystal to silver by donating electrons and the developer solution becomes oxidised. In this state the developer is not as active as the original solution, and so preservatives are added to help minimise the problem.

The pH range of the developer is from 9.6 to 10.4 and it is alkaline. Maintaining the alkalinity of the developer is important, so it is constantly being replenished with fresh developer solution from the replenishment tank.

A byproduct of the reaction which takes place during development is the production of hydrobromic acid which causes the developer to become less alkaline. This problem is overcome by adding a 'buffer' to maintain the pH to make sure the developer is working efficiently. If the activity of the developer falls there will be less contrast (see Chapter 3) on the final image when viewed.

A great advantage of PQ developers is their superadditivity. The activity produced when these two developers are combined is greater than if the two chemicals were added separately. The actual effect of the PQ developers is better than the expected activity. The reason for superadditivity is that the hydroquinone lessens the oxidation effect during development and it re-forms the by-products back into phenidone. The level of phenidone therefore does not get depleted so quickly; however, the hydroquinone level will still fall and need replenishment.

Buffer

Alkali is used to act as a 'buffer' and absorb hydrogen ions released during development to prevent the solution becoming more acidic. The chemicals which can be used are sodium carbonate and sodium bicarbonate.

As already mentioned, it is very important to maintain the correct level of alkalinity in the developer. The pH in the developer tank is usually 10.0 and in the replenishment tank 10.3. As pH is a log scale the activity of the solution in the replenishment tank is double that of the solution in the developer tank. A small difference in the pH level will affect the activity a great deal. The pH in the developer tank should be kept within + or − 0.2 of the accepted level. This can be checked by using a pH meter, which will measure the electrical potential of the solution. Another method is to use pH papers, but this is less accurate than using the pH meter.

Restrainer

The restrainer helps prevent the unexposed crystals from being developed, by increasing the effective barrier of the bromine ions. This improves the selectivity of the developer and reduces fog. The chemicals used are potassium bromide and with PQ developers an organic restrainer, called benzotriazole, is also required.

The 'starter solution', which is restrainer plus acetic acid, is added initially to developer solution when a fresh set of chemicals are put into a cleaned developer tank. If it is not added, it will cause a higher fog level on the image because the fresh developer solution will be very active. There is no restrainer in the replenisher tank.

Accelerator

The accelerator provides the correct pH level of the developer to keep it active so that it can be used efficiently. The chemicals necessary for this are sodium or potassium hydroxides.

Preservative

The developer reduces silver bromide to silver and therefore itself becomes oxidised. This is minimal compared with the amount of aerial oxidation of the developer, which means the developer solution oxidises in the atmosphere to form inert compounds. The aerial oxidation destroys the activity of the developer, and to try to prevent this happening a preservative is added to the developer solution. It is made up of chemicals such as sodium meta-bisulphite, sodium sulphite or potassium bisulphite.

Solvent

The solvent is water, and is a medium in which all the chemical reactions in the developer take place. It also helps the chemicals to penetrate the emulsion of the film. Some advantages of using water are that it is cheap and easily available. The main disadvantage is that water contains impurities such as calcium bicarbonates and sulphates, and magnesium bicarbonates and sulphates which 'harden' the water and make it less efficient as a solvent.

Sequestering agent

To 'soften' the water by reducing the impurities a sequestering agent is added. The chemical used is sodium salt of ethylene diamine tetra acetic acid (EDTA sodium salt).

Other additions to the developer solution

Hardening agent

During development the gelatin in the emulsion of the film swells. This agent is added to make the gelatin harder and give more protection to the film. However, it also causes the emulsion to absorb less of the developer chemicals, and to overcome this problem a wetting agent is used.

Wetting agent

This reduces the surface tension of the water around the film and allows more of the developer chemicals to penetrate the emulsion.

Anti-frothant

This will prevent the wetting agent from foaming.

Fungicide

Bacteria and fungi have a tendency to grow in the bottom of the development tank because of the warm temperature, and so fungicide is added to stop this happening.

COMPOSITION OF FIXER SOLUTION IN AN AUTOMATIC PROCESSOR

Acid

The acetic acid will stop further development of the image, and help to prevent unexposed crystals being developed. It also helps to maintain the correct pH level in the fixer solution, which is from 4.2 to 4.8, so that it works efficiently. Like the developer, the fixer solution is constantly being replenished by solution from the fixer replenishment tank. In theory the pH in the solution of the fixer tank and the solution of the replenisher tank are the same, but in practice generally the pH is higher (more alkaline) in the fixer tank solution.

Buffer

The chemicals which can be used as buffers are sodium acetate and acetic acid, and they help to maintain the level of pH in the fixer solution.

Fixing agent

The fixing agent is usually ammonium thiosulphate, and it causes the undeveloped crystals of silver bromide to be converted into a soluble solution so that they can be removed from the film. This gives the film archival properties, in other words, a permanent image that can be stored.

Preservative

During the fixing process sulphurisation occurs, which means sulphur is formed. This is because the thiosulphate in the fixer solution decomposes and it will make the fixer solution less efficient. To help prevent this a preservative is added such as sodium sulphite.

Hardener

If hardener is added to the fixer solution it makes the gelatin, in the emulsion of the film, less soft and helps prevent it swelling. The film dries more quickly and is less easily damaged when handled. The chemical used as a hardener is aluminium chloride or potassium sulphate.

Solvent

The solvent is water, and is a medium for the chemical reactions to take place in the fixer solution. It also helps dissolve any by-products.

HANDLING CHEMICALS

The developer and fixer solutions contain many corrosive chemicals. It is important, if these solutions are to be mixed by hand and put in the various tanks of the processors, that great care is taken.

It is advisable to read carefully the labels and instructions on all the bottles or cartons to be used. People who suffer from allergic conditions should be especially careful, as they probably have a more sensitive skin. Protective gloves, apron and glasses should be worn when mixing these solutions. If the chemicals do get in contact with the skin, rinse with plenty of water, and eyes should be flushed with water for at least ten minutes if they are affected. Medical advice should be sought as soon as possible. The place where the chemicals are mixed must be well ventilated, and there should be no food or drink allowed in that area.

The fixer solution and replenisher for the fix generally have two separate solutions with the correct amount of water to be added. The developer solution and replenisher have three separate solutions with the addition of water, but if fresh developer is made a fourth solution, 'starter solution', is included, which is not in the replenisher. It is vitally important that all the instructions, and the precautions to be taken, are read on the manu-facturer's leaflet.

Chemical mixers

The mixing of chemicals can be done automatically and accurately by chemical mixers which cost about £1000 (1985/6 prices). They have a capacity of 40 litres of each solution plus a reserve of 40 litres of the fixer and developer solutions, and give a warning signal when running out of chemicals. Although very efficient and time-saving they need to be used with an automatic processor with a reasonably large input of films, which is not always the case for radiotherapy departments.

AUTOMATIC PROCESSING

The exposed film is unloaded from the cassette either in a darkroom or using a daylight system (see Chapter 2). In the darkroom, with the safe-lights turned on, the film is placed on the feed tray, the widest part placed crossways to the correct edge of the tray. This is important for accurate replenishment rate of chemicals; however, some new processors take the surface area of the film into consideration so correct positioning of the film on the feed tray is less relevant. A delay is necessary before the next film is

Figure 4.2: Roller transport section. (Reproduced by permission of Kodak Ltd.)

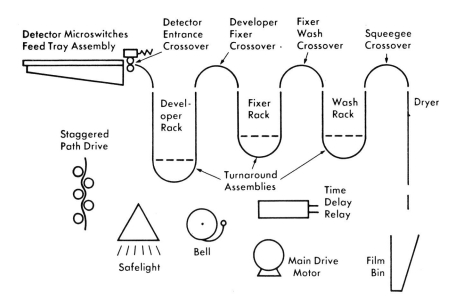

77

put through the processor, to prevent the films sticking together. Some units have a bell which sounds when it is safe to feed the next film.

When the film enters the processor a microswitch causes the rollers to start moving so that they will take up the film. This microswitch is also important for starting replenishment of the chemicals. The rollers have a staggered path drive and are offset to move the film more easily into the developer tank (see Figure 4.2).

Developer tank

The developer tank must have a constant temperature of about 30–32°C, to make sure the chemicals work efficiently. If the temperature becomes too high the films will become predominantly darker. The temperature is maintained by a heat exchanger and an associated heater with thermostat control.

There must be constant agitation to ensure the developer solution reaches all parts of the film. The agitation is caused by the recirculation pump which sucks out some developer solution, filters it and then the solution passes around the heater back to the developer tank (see Figure 4.3). The time taken for the film to go through the developer tank must be controlled; if it takes too long the films are over-developed and dark.

The processing cycle can be from 90 seconds up to eight minutes, depending on the type of film being used. Generally screen-type films have a short

Figure 4.3: Recirculation of developer. (Courtesy of Agfa Gevaert.)

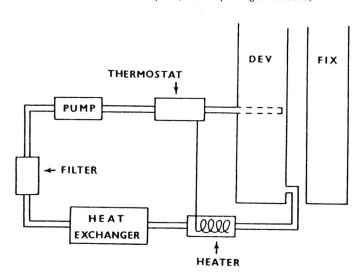

cycle but films which have a thicker emulsion, such as industrial films, need a longer cycle time. The film in an automatic processor, using a 90-second cycle, will take approximately 22 seconds to get through the developer tank.

The film is turned through 180° in the developer tank by the rollers, and then on to squeegee rollers. These are extremely important as they gently squeeze the film and remove excess developer. The squeegee rollers eliminate the need for a water rinse before the film enters the fixing solution. The film then passes through the cross-over assembly into the fixer tank (see Figure 4.2).

Fixer tank

This is situated between the wash tank and warm developer tank. It is import-ant that the fixer solution is recirculated to maintain agitation, so all parts of the film are fixed. If the processor is on a 90-second cycle, the film passes through the fixer tank in approximately 22 seconds.

Wash tank

The film has all its surplus chemicals removed in the wash tank. This takes about 22 seconds if the processor has a 90-second cycle time. The water is constantly circulated, up to 4–5 litres flowing per minute. To conserve water the modern processors sometimes use a cold-water spray which cuts the rate down to three litres per minute. In some processors the water flow is automatically switched off when there are no films being put through the processor. A certain amount of plumbing is required for the water flow.

Developer and fixer replenishment

The developer solution and fixer solutions need to be constantly replen-ished. This will maintain the pH levels to allow the chemicals to work effi-ciently, and ensure the correct level of the solution in the tanks (see Figure 4.4).

Drying system

The film must be dried so it can be easily handled. The temperature of the dryer is approximately 54′C. Hot air is forced through slits from tubes onto both sides of the film (see Figure 4.5). It is therefore important to site the processor carefully so that hot moist air can leave the system freely. If the processor has a 90-second cycle time the film is in the dryer for approximately 24 seconds. Some processors use infra-red lamps with cold-air blowers as a drying system. This uses less energy than the other type of system mentioned above, and therefore reduces operating costs.

The film then leaves the dryer and comes out into a receiver on the upper or lower part of the processor.

'Standby'

Another way of saving energy and water consumption is to have a 'standby' mode in the processor. This means the processor can be switched on ready for use, and when there are no films actually passing through it goes on 'standby'. When in 'standby' the dryer, water flow and main drive for the rollers are turned off, and only the systems for recirculation of developer and fixer solutions are left working.

MONITORING OF THE AUTOMATIC PROCESSOR

It is important for high-quality images that the processing cycle is correctly maintained and consistent in its performance.

Figure 4.4: Developer and fixer replenishment section. (Reproduced by permission of Kodak Ltd.)

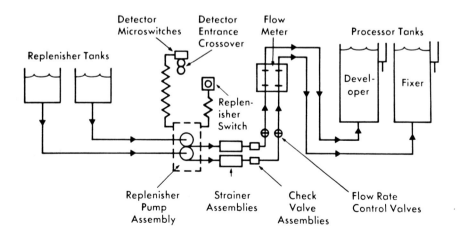

Figure 4.5: Drying system. (Courtesy of Agfa Gevaert.)

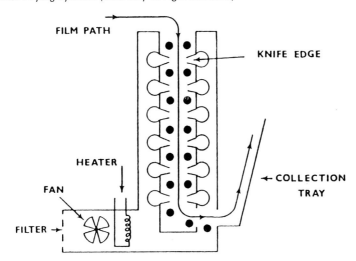

Sensitometric monitoring

The characteristic curve (see Chapter 3) shows the sensitometric properties of the film which include the effects of processing on the film. The shape of the curve will change slightly depending on, for instance, the temperature of the developer in the processor. Temperature increases will cause an increase in speed, average gradient and fog density (see Chapter 3) and these effects will show on the image. The change in the characteristic curve can be monitored and used to check that the processing of the films is being kept at the correct standard.[7]

Control strips

These are used to monitor the processor and are made by exposing X-ray film to a light sensitometer or by using a step wedge and ionising radiation (see Chapter 3). They can also be bought already prepared from the manufacturers; a box of 25 cost £18 (1985/6 prices).

The densities of the individual steps on the control strip are measured using a densitometer and a characteristic curve can be plotted (see Chapter 3). This can be used to find the film contrast, the speed and fog density of the film (see Chapter 3). However, in practice usually only the reference densities are used on a daily basis, and it is unnecessary to plot a characteristic curve every day.

Reference densities

There are three densities taken at certain steps which are noted on the control strip: a high density of 2, a low density of 1 and the fog density. These are called the reference densities. They are an indication of film contrast, which is the difference between the high and low reference densities, and the low reference density is an indicator of film speed.

The reference densities are found on the control strip and their daily variations plotted on a process control chart (see Figure 4.6). There is a certain amount of fluctuation allowed in the densities before action is taken on the processor.

Control limit

The control limit is the limit allowed for fluctuation where no action is taken. This is the area in between the dotted lines in Figure 4.6.

Action limit

The area in Figure 4.6 above the straight line is the action limit. Above this level it is considered necessary to check the processor.

Gross Fog

This should not exceed ± 0.05, as seen in Figure 4.6.

From the process control chart certain increases and decreases will indicate various problems of the processor.

Contrast and speed increase

This means the developer temperature may be too high. If a gradual increase is seen in the contrast and speed it could be due to over-replenishment of the developer, or could mean that the fixer solution is exhausted.

Contrast and speed decrease

The developer temperature may be too low. For a gradual decrease in speed and contrast it may mean under-replenishment of the chemicals.

Speed and fog increase, contrast decrease

The developer may contain fixer solution or the safe-lamps, if using a dark-room, may be incorrect or faulty.

Cross-over procedure

The control chart is only relevant for the same batch of film, and if there is no complete change in the processing chemicals. For a new batch of film or fresh chemicals a cross-over procedure should be used.

In the case of fresh chemicals, the old set of reference densities should be compared with a new set of reference densities. For new film, a few

Figure 4.6: Process control chart. (Reproduced by permission of Kodak Ltd.)

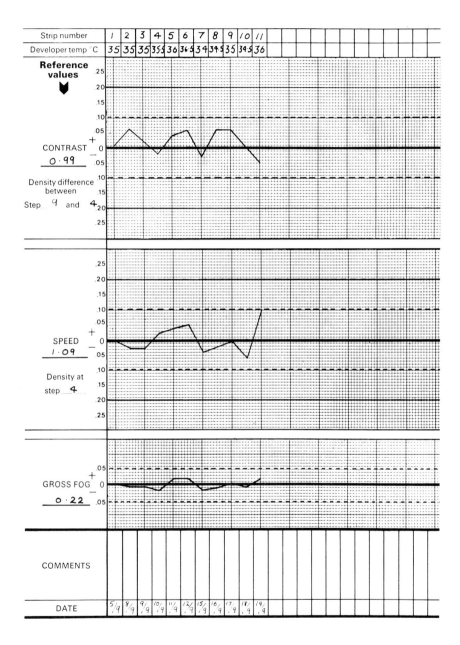

previous control strips should be processed with the new control strips and the reference densities noted for each type of film. If there is a great difference between the reference densities check the cross-over procedure again, the equipment used, such as the processor and densitometer, and the condition of the unexposed film used for the control strips. If the values are still widely different, the new set of reference densities should be used.

MAINTENANCE OF THE AUTOMATIC PROCESSOR

The processor should be switched off and isolated from the mains before any maintenance procedure is carried out.

Daily

The feed tray can be wiped and the wash tank drained. The cross-over rollers between the developer and fixer tanks should be sponged with water to remove all visible chemical deposits.

Weekly

Remove and clean the developer and fixer rollers.

Six-weekly

The developer and fixer solutions in the tanks should be completely changed and the tanks cleaned with water. In practice it is sometimes a longer interval.

Most manufacturers of processors recommend a 3-month or 6-month service.

TYPES OF AUTOMATIC PROCESSORS

Free-standing units

These are large units, for example, the Kodak RP X-OMAT model M8 with a height of 122 cm, width 83 cm and length 101 cm. This unit is capable of processing up to 250 films of 35 × 43 cm per hour, and has a 90-second cycle for processing the film, with temperatures controlled by thermostats and heaters. This processor has an automatic replenisher system which can be interfaced with a chemical mixer and silver recovery equipment (see later in this chapter). The model uses 3.8 litres of water per minute when processing films and the drier reaches temperatures up to 65°C. The use of a 'standby' mode is available which conserves water and energy. The cost of this equipment — including replenisher tanks, which are separate from the actual unit — is approximately £9800 (1985/6 prices).

This kind of processor is used in busy diagnostic departments and is probably unnecessary in a radiotherapy department, where the input of films is usually considerably lower than the diagnostic departments. However, the unit may be useful to radiotherapy departments if it is in an area where its facilities can be shared, to enable efficient use of such a processor.

Table-top automatic processors

As the name suggests, these can be placed on a table-top surface and are quite compact. The 3M XP505 model needs a maximum area of 0.62 square metres. The replenisher tanks, which are separate items, can be installed underneath the unit. It is a medium- to low-capacity processor; in other words, it will cope with handling a medium to small input of films. The processing cycle time is 90 seconds. To conserve energy and water there is a 'standby' mode and cold-water flow of 3 litres per minute. A certain amount of plumbing is required for the water flow when the model is installed. The dryer consists of infrared heaters, and cold air is blown around the films to dry them. This unit costs approximately £3950 (1985/6 prices).

A smaller version, which requires no plumbing, only a wall socket and replenishment containers (three 2.5-litre bottles, which are sited on top of the processor), is the Agfa Gevamatic 60. It is a low-capacity unit able to process 10–60 films per day. The processing cycle time is longer than the other table-top processor — about two minutes. It is a very economical unit costing £2570 (1985/6 prices), and there is no installation cost. It is easy to maintain and the manufacturers recommend cleaning the rollers once a fortnight, and a 2-month service if necessary. It has low electricity consumption and uses a small amount of water.

The table-top units are the more useful and economical type of processor for a radiotherapy department as they are small units, with low capacity and easy to maintain.

MANUAL PROCESSING

This system[6] is not in general use today, but some radiotherapy departments still have manual processors.

Chemicals

The developer and fixer chemicals used for manual processing are similar to the chemicals used in automatic processors, although for manual processing they are less active and diluted with more water. There is a slight difference, however, with some manual developer solutions as they do not contain hardener. The automatic processors have a hardener added to the developer, as well as the fixer solution, to help protect the film as it passes between the various rollers.

Processing

When using a manual processor the film is unloaded in the darkroom, under safe-light conditions, and clipped onto a hanger to make it secure. It is placed in the developer tank for 4–5 minutes at 20°C. The film must be agitated to prevent air bubbles forming on the emulsion, thus allowing even development. This movement also helps to disperse the by-products, bromine ions, or else the development of the emulsion will be inhibited. Then the film is placed in the rinse tank, containing water, for 20 seconds and agitated. This water must be changed daily if it is not running continuously.

Fixing of the film takes approximately ten minutes. It will clear and an image can be seen after 2–3 minutes; at this point it can be removed from the fix, but for archival purposes the film needs to be put back to completely fix for another 4–5 minutes. The film must be agitated when first placed in the fix and then left.

The wash tank can hold more than one film, and usually two or three are in the wash at the same time. On average the films should be left in the wash tank about 20 minutes. However, if there is a single film then only about ten minutes is needed. From the wash tank the film is drained and placed in a drying cabinet for 20 minutes.

A disadvantage of the manual system is that the whole process can take from 40 to 55 minutes. It is also difficult to standardise procedure to ensure each film is processed in exactly the same way. This system is slightly cheaper than an automatic processor. The cost of manual processing units varies from £1000 to £2000 (1985/6 prices).

Maintenance of the manual processor

On a daily basis all surfaces should be wiped clean, the water in the wash tank should be changed, unless it is continuously flowing, and developer and fixer solutions should be replenished. The developer solution should be completely changed every three months, and the fixer solution every 4–6 weeks. When changing the solutions the tanks should be drained and scrubbed with hot water before refilling.

SILVER RECOVERY

Silver is a natural resource, and the supply is diminishing rapidly as the demand, especially by the photographic industry, increases. It is economically viable to try to recover the silver from X-ray film and used fixer solutions. The reclaimed silver can be recycled, refined and re-used.

The market rate, which fluctuates on a day-to-day basis, will be paid per troy ounce of silver reclaimed. In 1980 the price of silver rocketed and the rate was £20 per troy ounce (approximately £640 per kg). There is now (1986) a more modest rate of £4.50 per troy ounce (approximately £144 per kg).

Another important reason for collecting used fix solution is to prevent the silver flowing down the drain and polluting the environment. This pollution occurs because the silver can cause harmful chemical reactions to occur with sewage.[8]

Amount of recoverable silver

Silver can be recovered from X-ray film and used fixer solution from the processor:

92 kg of used X-ray film produces 1 kg of silver;
200 litres of used fixer solution produces 1 kg of silver.

It is estimated that unused X-ray film has about seven grammes of silver per square metre. After exposure and processing about 40–50 per cent of this is left in the used fixer solution and the rest on the film.[9,10] However, with modern film emulsion technology the amount of silver in X-ray film has been reduced, and some unused X-ray films have only four grammes of silver per square metre.

The direct exposure film used in radiotherapy has a thick emulsion with a high silver content. When the film is used for verification of the treatment area usually only a small portion of the film is irradiated, and when processed a high yield of silver will be left in the used fixer solution.

It is required that X-rays are kept as a permanent record, and if storage becomes too bulky they can be sent to be microfilmed, in other words miniaturised, and the original X-ray films can then have their silver reclaimed. Any waste films must also be saved for silver recovery and must not be thrown away.

Solid waste containing silver

The silver can be recovered from discarded films by burning. The ashes are smelted with other substances into a molten material which separates out into the precious silver metal, and a lighter slag. The silver metal has impurities which are removed by a process called cupellation, and then electrolytically refined to form silver crystal. This is very close to 100 per cent pure silver, and it is melted down and made into bars which are stamped with the refiner's name, exact weight and serial number.

Silver refining is a very complicated process which needs to be done by specialists. They will buy the bulk product of solid waste containing the silver and the value will be known after refining.[9]

Fluid waste containing silver

There are a few different ways of obtaining silver from fluid waste and these are outlined below.

Bulk collection

The used fixer can be collected in containers and taken away at frequent intervals by the refiners. The amount of silver in the used fixer can be estimated 'on the spot' by using special test strips, and a price can be evaluated. The disadvantage is that this method of measuring the silver is not very accurate. The refiners will have to assay the silver before an exact price can be given.

Bulk collection is a convenient method of silver recovery, as the refiners are willing to collect small amounts of used fixer solution, which is an ideal situation for most radiotherapy departments.

Metal exchange

For this method of silver recovery a plastic pipe from the processor leads to a small polythene container, with a steel wool cartridge, and an outlet from the container to a convenient drain (see Figure 4.7). The waste fixer from the processor contains an acid solution, and when it is in contact with the steel wool cartridge in the container, the silver remains on the cartridge and the iron goes into solution.

The flow of the used fixer must be kept at the recommended speed by the manufacturer, or there will be poor metal exchange. It is also important the steel wool remains below the level of the fixer solution in the container, or oxidation will occur and rust will form. When the steel wool is completely exchanged it must be kept in the sealed container or else heat is generated and may eventually cause a fire.

This unit is easy to install, reliable, and requires little maintenance. It is approximately 95 per cent efficient at recovering the silver. Some refiners will collect the used steel wool cartridge and will replace with a new cartridge for a service fee of £30 (1986 price), but the actual equipment is supplied free of charge. The silver is reclaimed as for solid waste, and the silver content determined after refining.

The disadvantages of this kind of unit are that the level of the fixer must be checked regularly, and the efficiency of the unit drops after 60 per cent of the metal is exchanged. The fixer cannot be re-used after going through this unit, and the iron oxide which will flow into the drain with the exchanged fixer solution may cause a blockage.

Although more maintenance is involved with this method of silver recovery than with bulk collection, it is a cheap way of recovering the small amounts of silver which are produced from the used fixer solution in radio-therapy departments.

Electrolytic

The electrolytic method of silver recovery involves an electric current passing between two electrodes in a unit containing the used fixer solution. The anode electrode is made of carbon and the cathode electrode of stainless steel. When the current is switched on the silver will plate out onto the cathode and form silver flake. The fixer can then be recycled and used again in the main fixer tank of the processor — in practice, however, this generally does not happen. The silver flake is sent to the refiners to go through the refining process to become silver crystal and is eventually cast into pure silver bars. Electrolytic silver recovery is about 98 per cent efficient at reclaiming silver from the used fixer.

High current density units

Tradenames such as 'Silver King' or 'Silvamatic' refer to high current density units which are needed for this method of silver recovery. The used

Figure 4.7: Typical metal exchange units. (Courtesy of John Betts Refiners Ltd.)

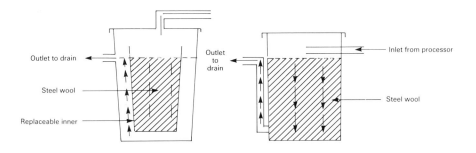

fixer solution is agitated by a rotating cathode and anode and by pumping air through the solution. This allows a high intensity of current to be used, up to about 21 amps, which means a rapid recovery of silver. The output of silver per hour can be up to 100 grammes. The most modern units are computer-controlled and have a sensing device which can compensate for the variations of silver content in the used fixer. If the silver content is too low sulphide can be formed on the cathode, preventing efficient plating. These units are sealed and no fumes are given off. There is a lockable head for security reasons, as silver is a valuable commodity.

High current density units are very efficient and are used with automatic processors which have a large output of used fixer solution. The cost of the equipment ranges from £600 to £1650 per unit (1985/6 prices).

Tailing unit

One of the most efficient methods of recovering silver from used fixer solution is by using a tailing unit. This system consists of a high current density unit, with a metal exchange unit taking the outflow of the fixer which has just been through the electrolytic unit. For this method to be effective a large quantity of used fixer is required.

THE DARKROOM

The darkroom,[11,12] when used to handle X-ray film, must be a light-tight area to prevent fogging the sensitive emulsion of the film. To ensure that there is no external light entering the darkroom all the lights are turned off in the darkroom for 10 minutes, and any stray light will be seen. It is essential to use the correct safelights (see later in this chapter) so as not to impair the image. The walls of the darkroom should be painted a light colour, to give the greatest amount of reflection from the safelights.

The construction of the darkroom should be solid and the walls, the floor and the ceiling should have adequate protection from ionising radiation to prevent fogging of the film. It is important to have good ventilation and fresh airflow with a filter to remove dust particles and a working temperature of 18–20°C.

A rectangular darkroom is more useful, as it is unnecessary to have a great amount of central floor space. When using an automatic processor a minimum height of three metres is required, and seven square metres floor space. However, some automatic processors are sited so that only the feed tray is in the darkroom and the rest of the processor is outside against the adjoining wall. A manual processing unit needs more space for comfortable working: ten square metres and a height of three metres.

The manual processor has a 'wet' and 'dry' bench in the darkroom and each area should be kept as designated. The automatic processor requires only a dry bench in the darkroom. The work bench should not be covered with any kind of plastic, as this will cause static electricity; a linoleum is preferred.

All surfaces in the darkroom should be cleaned regularly to remove dust and dirt as this will help prevent damage to the films, screens and cassettes. The floor should be covered with non-slip, waterproof material, such as vinyl sheeting, which if curved slightly up the walls, will stop liquid getting underneath the floor covering. Plumbing and electrical supplies for the processor should be from the manufacturer's specifications.

Some films can be stored in the darkroom, in a drawer or hopper which must be light-tight even when the room lights are turned on, but the main film store should be away from the darkroom.

SAFELIGHTS

Safelights[13,14] are used in the darkroom to allow X-ray film to be handled without fogging the film. It is important the correct filter is used in the safe-lamp, so that the only light emitted from the lamp is that to which the film is not sensitive. For a blue-sensitive film an orange safelight is acceptable, but for a green-sensitive film a red filter is needed in the safelight.

Direct illumination

This implies that the light from the safelight is falling directly onto the film. When using the correct filter, the safelight can be 1.2 metres away from the working surface where the film is being handled.

Indirect illumination

The light from the safelight is reflected from the walls or ceiling in the darkroom to give general illumination.

There are various types of safelights: wall-mounted and cone-shaped, suspended from the ceiling and square, and in the form of long fluorescent tubes. Some processors have a safelight over the feed tray which is automatically switched off when feeding the film.

The wall-mounted lamp with the correct colour filter should have a 15 or 25 watt bulb. If the wattage of the bulb is too high it may cause fogging of the film and damage the filter. The square safelight from the ceiling usually has two filters, the bottom filter red for direct illumination and the top filter orange for indirect illumination. The cost of the lamps and filters depends on the type and size required and ranges from £40 to £65 (1985/6 prices).

Maintenance

It is important that the filter in any safelight can be identified when the

Figure 4.8: Test device for safelight test. (Reproduced by permission of Kodak Ltd.)

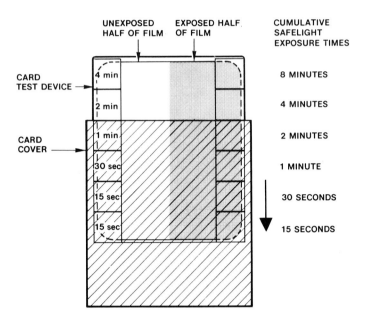

lamp is viewed directly. The safelights and filters should be regularly cleaned with a damp cloth to remove dust. They must be checked for any kind of damage as this may cause fogging on the film. The filters can fade after three years, and to ensure efficiency a test can be performed.

Safelight test

This is performed to check that the safelight and filter[12] being used is not fogging the films, when exposed and unexposed film are being handled in the darkroom. The fastest film which is used should be tested as a faster film is more sensitive to light.

Test device

A sheet of card larger than the film is needed. With the longer edges a flap of about 3 cm is made on each side, so that the X-ray film can slot inside, as shown on Figure 4.8. Divide the flaps into equal portions of six and write the following times on each flap: 4 min, 2 min, 1 min, 30 s, 15 s and 15 s as in Figure 4.8.

Expose the film to a density between 0.5 and 1.0 (see Chapter 3) and protect one half of the film with lead. Unload the film in total darkness, in the darkroom, and put the film into the test device. Place a large card over the top to completely cover the film. Switch on the safelight then gradually uncover the card as recommended by the times on the flap. The top portion is exposed for a total of eight minutes and the last part for 15 seconds. The safelight is now switched off and the film processed in total darkness.

Inspect the developed film and using a densitometer (see Chapter 3) find the areas on the film and under the flap which only differ by a density of 0.05. Do this for both the exposed and unexposed parts of the film. The time can then be determined in which the film can be safely handled without fogging. In practice, for a safety margin, the handling time should be shorter than this. The test can be carried out if the safelighting is thought to be faulty, or at 6-month or yearly intervals.

HANDLING X-RAY FILM

Great care should be taken when handling X-ray film in the darkroom as it is very sensitive to light and pressure, especially after the film has been exposed to radiation. Film handling time in the darkroom has been reduced because of the use of automatic processors. There is therefore less chance of damaging the film, or fogging the image.

To unload a cassette

Ensure the safelights are turned on, the main lights turned off and the darkroom is locked. The catch or clips are released on the cassette and then this side of the cassette is placed down on to the bench. Open the cassette, and angle the other side of the cassette towards the bench to tip out the exposed film. Carefully hold the film as it drops forward at a corner or the edge. Lift the film out of the cassette and take the opposite edge of the film with the other hand and place in the feed tray of the automatic processor, or clip into a hanger for manual processing.

To load a cassette

Place the side without any catches or clips flat onto the bench. Open the cassette and carefully place the film into the cassette by touching only the edge or corners of the film, and then secure the cassette.

Packing

There are several different ways of packing X-ray film.

Ready pack

The film is contained in a light-tight envelope which has been heat-sealed. Inside the envelope the film is within a folder of yellow paper. Generally there are 50 films in a box. The film can be used directly and does not need to be loaded into a cassette in the darkroom. This kind of packaging makes the film more expensive.

Interleaved

Each separate sheet of film is covered by a folder of yellow paper. Although the paper will help protect the film during storage and handling it can cause marks which appear on the image when processed. It is necessary that the film is loaded into a cassette in the darkroom, under safe-light conditions. There can be 100 sheets in a box, and because of the special packing it is more costly than non-interleaved film, but less expensive than 'ready pack' film.

Non-interleaved

The separate sheets of film are not surrounded by yellow paper. The film needs to be loaded into a cassette. There can be 100 films in a box or two packs of 50 films in heat-sealed foil pouches.

Compact packaging

This consists of heat-sealed pouches containing 100 films in each pouch with stiffeners for rigidity, and five pouches in a carton. This compact packaging saves storage room; at least a 28 per cent saving of space is quoted by the manufacturer. The pouches can be stored and used individually.

Storage

Film should be stored away from the darkroom and it will become fogged unless protected from light and ionising radiation. If the film is to be stored for about two months then it is necessary to keep it at a temperature of 18°C and a relative humidity of 50–60 per cent. For periods longer than two months the temperature must be lower than 15°C with a 50–60 per cent humidity or the film will deteriorate. When the film is taken out of the cool storage it should be allowed to reach room temperature gradually, to prevent condensation.

The boxes of film should be placed vertically as film is sensitive to pressure; if stored horizontally the bottom layers may become damaged. The processing chemicals should not be in the same store room as the film in case fumes are given off, which may cause a variation in the quality of the film. If the film is used after the expiry date it may be slightly fogged and give a poor image. It is important to rotate stock and to try to use the older films first.

VIEWING OF THE IMAGE

Good viewing conditions are essential to show the final image off to its best advantage. The viewing boxes or illuminators must have a uniform intensity of light across the surface of the viewing area,[13] otherwise the assessment of the image may be altered.

The recommended viewing distance is 40 cm to allow a good response from the eye. The lighting in the area, where viewing of the image takes place, should be subdued to help prevent glare. If a bank of viewing boxes is used, and all illuminated at the same time, it may be necessary to mask part of the film or just use one viewing box because of the glare from the other illuminators. The X-ray film is made with a blue-tinted base which also helps to stop the glare from the viewing box. If the image on the film is very dark, which is quite often the case for radiotherapy verification films, an intense bright light is needed. This can be a single lamp or a small area at the side of the viewing box.

Depending on the type, and whether a bank of viewing boxes is required, the cost of the viewing equipment varies from £60 to £1200 (1985/6 prices).

FILM FAULTS

The following text describes a few examples of film faults. For more details see Chesney and Chesney, and Jenkins, in Further Reading.

High-density marks

These will show as darker areas on the viewed image after processing.[15]

If the film is splashed with developer before being processed, this area will develop more quickly and leave a dark splash mark on the film. If any water gets onto the film before processing it causes the emulsion to soften, and the area will again develop more quickly, so dark fingerprints are seen when the film is handled with wet hands. If the film is handled too tightly it will cause high-density marks, as the pressure on the emulsion allows it to be developed more easily in those areas and can leave crescent-shaped marks. Dark lines on the film may be the result of uneven transit through the rollers of an automatic processor.

Static electricity will appear as branched lines on the film (see Figure 4.9). The build-up of static can be caused in the darkroom by a 'Formica'-covered bench, dry atmosphere, nylon clothing being worn by handler or the continual loading and unloading of the cassette with film. It can be reduced by having a linoleum top for the bench, good airflow in the darkroom and regular cleaning of screens in the cassettes with an anti-static cleaner.

Fogging will occur if a box of films is opened in white light by mistake; the ends of the films will have dark edges when they are processed. The film can also be fogged by certain chemicals such as lead-based paint, formaldehyde, carbon monoxide and mercury. The background radiation must be below a certain level or films will be fogged, so thought must be given to the construction of the darkroom or film store, especially if using granite or breeze blocks.

Figure 4.9: Film fault caused by static electricity.

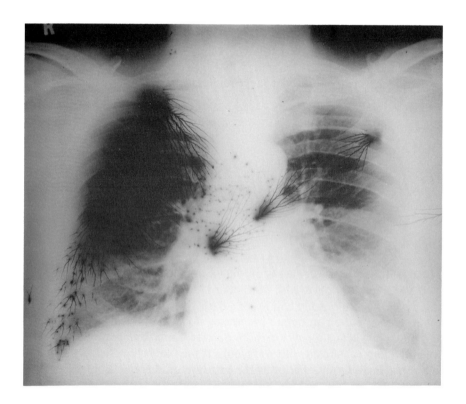

Low-density marks

These will show as light-coloured marks on the processed image.[15]

If fixer solution is splashed onto a film before developing, the silver is removed in that area, and will show as a light mark. When the film is not fixed for long enough it will have a white stain and if not adequately washed, after a period of storage, a brown stain will be seen.

With bad handling of the film, pressure marks such as fingerprints can show as light-coloured marks. If the handler has oily or greasy hands this will act as a barrier to developer and show as light areas. The cassettes or screens could be damaged and some areas may show low-density marks on the film. This will be easily recognised as the marks will always be in the same place on different films.

Dichroic fog

This is a generalised fault when developer is carried over into the fixer, but rarely happens nowadays because of the efficient automatic processors. The film will have a pink tinge when viewed with transmitted light and appear slightly green in colour with reflected light.

REFERENCES

1. James, T.H. (1977) *The Theory of the Photographic Process*, 4th edn., Macmillan, London, pp. 1–77, 88–145, 645, 673.
2. Agfa Gevaert, 'The formation of the latent image', technical literature.
3. Meredith, W.J. and Massey, J.B. (1977) *Fundamental Physics of Radiology*, 3rd edn, Wright, Bristol, pp. 166–74.
4. Agfa Gevaert, 'Photochemistry of automatic processors', technical literature.
5. Jenkins, D. (1980) *Radiographic Photography and Imaging Processes*, MTP Press, Lancaster, pp. 190–221.
6. Kodak, 'X-ray recording materials', *Fundamentals of Radiographic Photography*, vol. II, pp. 40–6.
7. Kodak, 'Image quality control', *Fundamentals of Radiographic Photography*, vol. I, pp. 27–37.
8. Agfa Gevaert, 'Hints for a better environment', technical literature, pp. 6–7.
9. John Betts Refiners Ltd, 'Recovering silver from medical resources', technical literature.
10. Eastman Kodak Company (1979) 'Recovering silver from photographic materials', technical literature, pp. 6–12.
11. Kodak, 'X-ray recording materials', *Fundamentals of Photography*, vol. II, pp. 35–7.
12. Kodak, 'Radiographic quality', *Fundamentals of Photography*, vol. III, pp. 49–53.
13. Jenkins, D. (1980) *Radiographic Photography and Imaging Processes*, MTP Press, Lancaster, pp. 177–80, 161–5.

14. Hurtgen, T.P. (1978) 'Safelights in the automated darkroom', *Medical Radiography and Photography*, vol. 54, no. 2.
15. Agfa Gevaert, 'Diagnosing film faults', technical literature.

Private communications

T. Cropper (Marketing Education Centre, Kodak); B. Turner; M. Lovegrove; D. Rothery (3M); N. Smith (Agfa Gevaert); B. Turner.

Manufacturers' literature

Agfa Gevaert Diagnostic Imaging Systems Medical Division, Price List April 1985.
Agfa Gevaert, 60 Gevamatic.
Du Pont, Cronex T6.
Du Pont, Close to perfection, Cronex T5A.
Du Pont, Cronex Automatic Chemical Mixer.
John Betts Refiners Ltd, Silvamatic Electrolytic Silver Recovery Equipment, JBR MK8 Silver Recovery Unit.
Kodak, Medical Buyers Guide to the DHSS, April 1985.
3M, XP505 and XP510/6 X-ray Film Processors.
3M, Storage of Photographic Products.
May and Baker, Matalex Developer System, Fixaplus Fixer System, Perfix High Speed Manual X-ray Fixer and Polycon Variable Contrast Manual X-ray Developer.

FURTHER READING

Chesney, D.N. and Chesney, M.O. (1981) *Radiographic Imaging*, 4th edn, Blackwell Scientific Publications, Oxford, pp. 232–8.
Gifford, D. (1984) *A Handbook of Physics for Radiologists and Radiographers*, John Wiley and Sons, Chichester, pp. 198–203.
James, T.H. (1977) *The Theory of the Photographic Process*, 4th edn, Macmillan, London.
Jenkins, D. (1980) *Radiographic Photography and Imaging Processes*, MTP Press, Lancaster, pp. 295–7.

5

The Simulator — Equipment

The simulator is needed for a radiotherapy department to produce an image of a treatment field area in relation to surface markings on a patient. It is important that the simulator is like the treatment unit in design such as beam collimation, gantry and couch so that a reproducible 'set-up' can be achieved (see Figure 5.1). This unit is combined with a diagnostic X-ray tube to enable useful images to be taken which have good definition (see Chapter 3).

It is possible for other types of equipment to do a similar job, such as a mobile X-ray unit or a DXR treatment unit with a voltage setting around 125 kV, but each has its own problems as regards simulating a treatment area or producing a useful image. This chapter will deal with the actual equipment details of the simulator, and the use of the simulator will be described in Chapter 6.

SPECIFICATIONS OF A SIMULATOR

The simulator is made up of two systems: an X-ray system and a mechanical system.

X-ray system

This consists of an X-ray tube, X-ray generator and X-ray image intensifier system.

Mechanical system

This consists of a gantry and stand, collimator, couch and local and remote control.

The following text will expand on each of these components of the simulator.

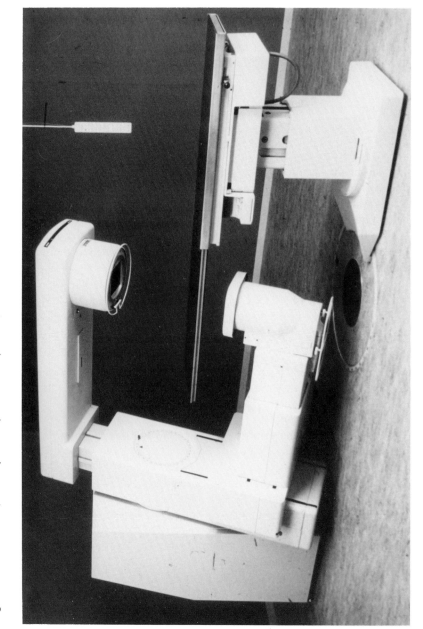

Figure 5.1: Simulator. (Courtesy of Philips Medical Systems.)

X-ray tube

There are two main kinds of X-ray tubes — the stationary anode and the rotating anode tube. The latter (see Figure 5.2) is preferred for the simulator because it is able to withstand more power without being damaged. The cost of a rotating anode tube will vary from £5000 to £8000 (1986/7 prices). An X-ray tube is made up of a cathode and an anode.

Cathode

The cathode assembly contains a filament which is a coil of tungsten wire. When heated to very high temperatures this gives off electrons by thermionic emission. The cathode can have two different-size filaments to form a large or small stream of electrons, which will give a broad or fine focus X-ray beam.[1] The broad focus will allow a higher rating to be used (see below) and the fine focus will reduce unsharpness (see Chapter 3).

The flow of electrons from the cathode to the anode is the tube current, and the average tube current is measured in mA. The total electron flow is the mA × time for the exposure, and is measured in mAs.

Anode

The stream of electrons is directed at the target on the anode,[2] by the focusing cup of the cathode structure. Electrons are pulled towards the anode when it has a positive potential with respect to the cathode. The positive potential is the peak kilovoltage (kVp) and is the maximum instantaneous kilovoltage at any time during the exposure.

The electrons from the filament strike the target and X-rays are produced at the focal spot.

Focal spot

The area of the target bombarded by the electrons is called the actual or real focal spot. The effective or apparent focal spot is the actual focal spot area projected down at right angles, and gives the size which manufacturers refer to as the focal spot (see Chapter 3). The smaller the effective focal spot the less unsharpness produced on the image (see Chapter 3). The X-ray tube for the simulator can have a fine focus or focal spot of 0.3–0.6 mm^2 and a broad focus of 0.7–1.2 mm^2.

X-ray production

This is inefficient in an X-ray tube, and only 1 per cent of X-rays are

Figure 5.2: Rotating anode tube and casing. (Reproduced by permission of E. Forster and MTP Press Ltd.)

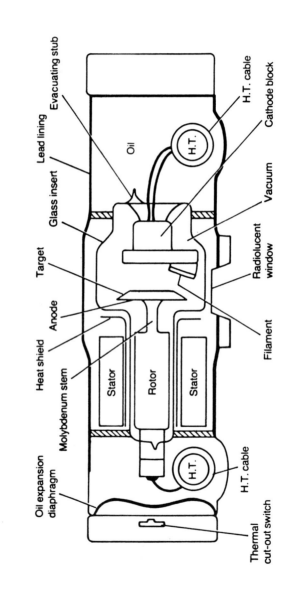

produced with about 95–99 per cent heat. It is important that the heat is removed so that no damage is sustained by the equipment. The rotating anode removes heat mainly by radiation. The anode is rotated at high speed, 9000 rpm preferred for the simulator,[3] and it reaches white-hot temperatures. At this level the removal of heat by radiation from the anode is extremely efficient.[4]

Target

This is generally made from a tungsten–rhenium alloy, and in more modern tubes the target disc has slits across it to allow for expansion and contraction without distorting. Sometimes a compound target is used — rhenium–tungsten alloy backed by molybdenum or graphite — which will allow a higher rating (see below). This is because the compound target can withstand more heat before it is damaged than the usual type of target.[5] The size of the target commonly used with the simulator is from 8 to 10 cm in diameter.

Target angle

The target is angled slightly to enable a reasonable-sized beam of X-rays to be produced. An angle such as 20° will allow larger areas to be imaged than a steeper angle of 7°. However, the larger angle will cause more unsharpness of the image than the smaller angle (see Chapter 3).

Anode heel effect

There is a reduction of intensity of the X-rays produced at approximately the same angle as the target. This is because they are attenuated by the target material, and this is called the anode heel effect.[6] The effect is reduced for larger angles of the anode which will give a more even intensity across the beam, and help prevent the anode side of the image being paler or less dense.

A compromise is made for the simulator and the target angle is usually between 12° and 16°, which allows a large field size to be imaged, with a reasonably homogeneous beam and an acceptable amount of unsharpness.

Tube insert

The anode and cathode of the X-ray tube are mounted in a glass envelope, usually borosilicate glass, which encloses a vacuum. This structure is called the tube insert. The glass provides electrical insulation to prevent an electrical current flowing out through the tube insert.

At high temperatures evaporation of the filament can occur which deposits a thin layer of tungsten on the glass insert and acts as a third electrode. This layer can draw away some of the electrons which should be directed towards the anode, and will damage the glass insert. The Philips Localizer Simulator uses a Rotalix X-ray tube, and the tube insert has a central portion made of steel with glass at the anode end and ceramic at the cathode end.[7] The central metal part of the Rotalix tube will attenuate stray electrons so that higher temperatures can be tolerated by the tube. This means it will have a better rating than the conventional type of X-ray tubes.

Tube housing

The housing surrounds the tube insert and provides a high-voltage terminal necessary to convey the energy for the exposure. It acts as a shield against stray radiation as it is lead-lined except at the radiolucent window (see Figure 5.2). It is filled with oil to provide insulation and convect heat away from the tube insert.

There is a diaphragm of oil-resistant synthetic rubber at one end of the housing (see Figure 5.2) which acts as a safety device. As the area around the tube insert becomes hot, heat is convected into the surrounding oil. The oil expands and if the temperature becomes too high the diaphragm will operate a contact and prevent further working of the equipment. Some simulators have an air circulator fitted to the outside of the tube housing in the form of a small fan. This increases the air flow around the tube and doubles the cooling rate of the X-ray tube.

The tube housing allows precise positioning of the tube insert so that the focal spot can be aligned accurately with the collimator system. This is to make sure that the centre of the X-ray beam is coincident with the centre of the optical light beam.

Inherent filtration

The very low-energy X-rays are not useful for the production of the image. The X-ray tube insert, oil and radiolucent window which forms the inherent filtration, absorb a small amount of the low-energy radiation from the X-ray beam. It is also necessary to add extra filtration at the X-ray window to ensure most of the low-energy radiation is absorbed. The total filtration should not be less than 1.5 mm aluminium for voltages up to 70 kV, 2.00 mm aluminium from 70 to 100 kV and then 0.1 mm per kV above 100 kV.[7] The removal of these low-energy X-rays also helps to reduce the patient's skin dose.

RATING

The rating of the X-ray tube is important, and it establishes values which, from the manufacturer's experience and calculations, provides the equipment with a long life.

A definition of rating is the combination of exposure settings which the unit can withstand without incurring unacceptable damage. There will be general wear and tear on the unit during everyday usage, such as the anode becoming pitted and the filament slightly thinner, but a level could be reached which will produce damage to the tube and effectively reduce its life.

A short exposure at very high mA may damage the anode by melting the focal area; alternatively, an extremely long exposure at low mA may cause overheating and damage to the anode or housing. These examples are of single exposures. Another problem can occur with multiple exposures: if there is not sufficient cooling time between exposures a great deal of damage can be caused to the anode.

To help reduce the risk of damage to the equipment the manufacturers supply rating charts with X-ray tubes. Each chart is relevant only for the specified tube and the certain factors which can be selected — such as broad focus, fine focus, kVp, mAs and for single or multiple exposures.[8] There are basically two types of rating charts — electrical and thermal.

Electrical rating charts

Rating for single exposure

A rating chart is shown in Figure 5.3, and any exposures under the line are within safe limits but above the line unacceptable damage is caused to the X-ray tube. A logarithm scale is used because of the wide range of exposure times.

Rating chart for broad and fine focus

The rating charts for the broad and fine focus are shown in the simplified diagram (see Figure 5.4). The rating for the fine focus is lower than that for the broad focus because the electron beam is focused on a smaller area for a fine focus, therefore more heat is produced for the same mA. The charts also show that as the kVp is increased smaller values of mA must be given. The reason is that as the kVp increases the energy of the electrons increases. Because of this greater energy the number of electrons must be reduced so that the anode does not become too hot. It is therefore necessary to lower the mA.

Thermal rating charts

For multiple exposures it is important to use thermal rating charts such as the anode cooling curve and the anode heating curve.[8,9]

Figure 5.3: Rating chart. (Courtesy of Picker International Ltd.)

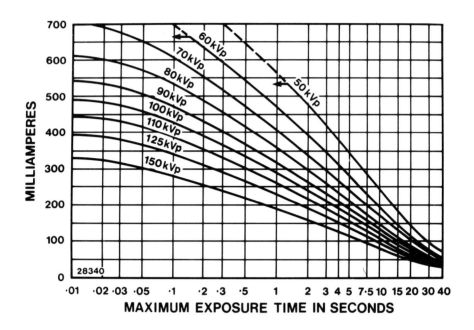

Anode cooling curve

If the exposures are too close together this does not give the anode time to cool down. The cooling curve shows how a combination of exposures are within the safety limits. The unit of measurement of this energy is the heat unit (HU) and it is kVp × mA × seconds for single-phase equipment (see below) and when three-phase equipment is used (see below), energy is quoted in joules, which is also kVp × mA × seconds.

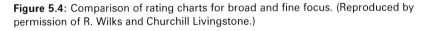

Figure 5.4: Comparison of rating charts for broad and fine focus. (Reproduced by permission of R. Wilks and Churchill Livingstone.)

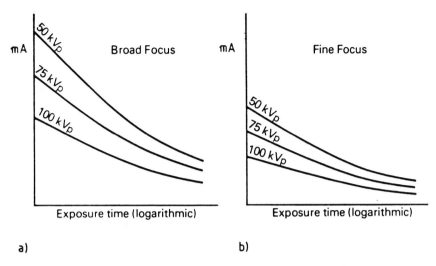

a)   b)

The chart in Figure 5.5 shows that the anode has a maximum heat storage capacity of 80,000 HU. This means that it is not desirable to operate the X-ray tube above this level. In the simple diagram if an exposure is given which produces 40,000 HU (point P) it then takes five minutes for the anode to cool down to 20,000 HU (point Q). If multiple exposures are needed it is possible to add the heat units produced together, with reference to the time interval, and by using the cooling curve check that the rating is not exceeded.

Anode heating curve

When long exposures are used, such as in fluoroscopy (screening), the anode heats up initially and then reaches thermal equilibrium. This means the rate of heat generated by the electron beam is balanced by the rate of heat lost from the anode.

In Figure 5.6 this particular anode has a maximum heat storage capacity of 100,000 HU; above this level unacceptable damage is incurred at the anode. The chart (see Figure 5.6) shows that an exposure which causes 1000 HU per second will exceed the rating, 500 HU per second will level off at the maximum value and 100 HU per second will produce the thermal equilibrium at a much lower acceptable level.

In practice the anode cooling curve and heating curve can be on the same graph.

Interlocks

Most X-ray units have interlocks installed to prevent overloading, but only

107

Figure 5.5: Anode cooling curve. (Reproduced by permission of R. Wilks and Churchill Livingstone.)

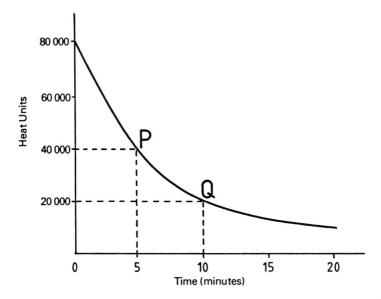

allow protection for single exposures and not multiple exposures. However, some of the more modern units do take into account the heat accumulation, and have interlocks which protect from overloading when using multiple exposures.

X-RAY GENERATOR

The X-ray generator receives power from the main generating system which it uses to attain the high voltages needed to produce X-rays. The conventional type of generators consist of a power cabinet, high-tension transformer tank with high-tension cables, and a control console. Nowadays, with the use of new technology and microprocessor elements, a much slimmer high-tension transformer can be made which needs far less room than the older generators.

X-ray circuits

These are within the various parts of the generator and are basically a primary circuit and a secondary circuit. The primary circuit is at low tension from the mains, 240 or 415 volts. The secondary circuit is at high

Figure 5.6: Anode heating curve. (Reproduced by permission of R. Wilks and Churchill Livingstone.)

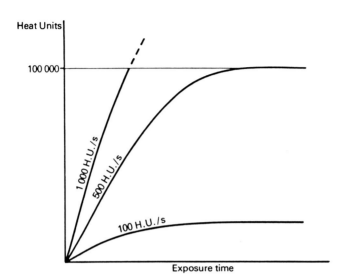

tension, for instance at 75 kVp, depending on the exposure required for the image.

Primary circuit

This contains main switches, fuses, circuit-breakers, autotransformer, line voltage compensator, kV selector, pre-reading kV meter, primary winding of high-tension transformer, timer circuit, filament transformer and stabiliser.

Secondary circuit

This has the secondary winding of the high-tension transformer, high-tension rectifiers, secondary winding of filament transformer and X-ray tube.

The equipment in the primary and secondary X-ray circuit will not be explained in this book; for further information see References 10 and 11.

X-ray generators can be either single-phase two-pulse, three-phase six-pulse or twelve-pulse, constant potential or the newer multi-pulse units. The difference in these types of generators depends on the supply from the mains and the type of rectification in the X-ray circuit of the generator.

Rectification

An alternating supply (AC) is used from the mains to the X-ray generator.[12,13] This is so that voltages can be stepped up and down to the correct level for use in the different transformers in the X-ray circuit. Rectification is needed to simulate a steady high voltage with direct current (DC) to keep the cathode at a negative potential and the anode at a positive potential for efficient generation of X-rays.

Single-phase, two-pulse

This type of generator uses a single-phase supply[12] from the mains, which means each cycle is made up of a positive and a negative peak, and it has four rectifiers. The rectifiers are in the form of diode valves[11] or solid-state rectifiers, and allow the current to pass in one direction only, so that the cathode is always negative and the anode positive.

This type of rectification allows the negative peak of the cycle to be used for X-ray production as well as the positive peak. The disadvantage is that, as the voltage continually drops and then reaches a maximum, the energy of the X-rays being produced is not constant.

Three-phase, six-pulse or twelve-pulse

The generator requires a three-phase supply from the mains, a cycle containing three positive and three negative peaks.[13] Six or twelve rectifiers are used in the X-ray circuit and produce a system which is in effect similar to a constant DC voltage, but with a slight 'ripple', across the X-ray tube.

The advantage is that more X-rays are produced than with the single-phase system for a similar exposure because the voltage is not pulsating.[11] The X-rays generated are of better quality than for single-phase, and less low-energy radiation is produced, which means a lower skin dose to the patient. A higher mA can be supplied with three-phase supply and therefore exposure times can be reduced. This means less unsharpness of the image as the blurring caused by involuntary movement is minimal (see Chapter 3).

Constant potential

The rectified circuits already mentioned give a slight pulsating voltage ('ripple' effect). This can be smoothed by adding capacitors and triodes to the secondary circuit,[12] and the generator will then produce a constant potential.

Multi-pulse

This is a newer concept and can be used with a single- or three-phase supply from the mains. It will generate a near-constant potential voltage and, the manufacturers suggest, with an even better gain of X-ray production than for the conventional type of generator.

The multi-pulse generator has the usual type of rectification as for a two-pulse or six-pulse system, and then a frequency converter changes the frequency (mains supply 50 Hz UK, 60 Hz USA) up to 10 kHz.[11] This is then rectified again, smoothed with capacitors and a near-constant potential voltage capable of high intensity is produced.

Power of the generator

This is defined with different units for single-phase and three-phase because of the pulsating voltage of single-phase and the near-constant potential of three-phase.

Single-phase power is quoted in HU/s
$$HU/s = kVp \times mA$$
Three-phase power is quoted in joules/s = watts
$$watts = kVp \times mA$$
An approximate conversion of HU /s to watts is HU/s $\times$ 0.7

Single-phase generators can achieve medium to high power outputs, 25 to 80 kW, and the three-phase units high power outputs from 50 to 200 kW. The multi-pulse generators at present produce outputs from 30 to 100 kW. The more powerful the generator the more costly is the unit, and the prices range from £16,000 to £46,000 (1986/7 prices).

Rating of the generator

This is important, as it will show the variation of maximum exposures which can be used without damaging the equipment. A generator with an 80 kW output, for example, may give 1000 mA at 80 kVp, 800 mA at 100 kVp but only 500 mA at 150 kVp (75 kW) which shows that at higher kV the generator can only withstand a lower mA.[13]

The generator for the simulator should be capable of 500 mA at 90 kVp and 300 mA at 150 kVp to ensure useful radiographs, and for screening 10 mA at 125 kV.[14] However, most modern simulators have generators which exceed these limits; for instance the Varian Ximatron CX has a three-phase, six-pulse generator, maximum output of 75 kW, with a rating

111

of 700 mA at 100 kVp, 600 mA at 125 kVp and for screening 20 mA at 120 kV.

Control console

The X-ray generator controls the exposure needed for a static image and the exposure for fluoroscopy (screening). (The exposure is made up of kV, mA and time.) It has a control console which allows the appropriate factors to be chosen for an exposure.

The basic control panel has switches, or nowadays, smooth touch control, for kV, mA and time or mAs with their various read-outs and for broad or fine focus. A more sophisticated set such as a three-phase, twelve-pulse generator includes a computer program which relates to parts of the body and a pre-set automatic exposure can be given.

The exposure button is at the end of a short cable, and to make the exposure the button is slightly depressed. This puts the unit into 'prep', or preparation, and there is a short delay before the exposure can be given. This allows time for the filament of the X-ray tube to attain the correct temperature and the anode to reach full rotational speed. The unit should be held in 'prep' for as short a time as possible to prolong the life of the filament. When the exposure is made a warning light on the console will illuminate.

An on/off button or control will turn the unit on and off from the mains. The more modern units will automatically compensate for mains fluctuations but for the older units this is done manually and there is a line voltage compensator dial and control.

The controls for fluoroscopy are on a separate part of the console. The settings will show kV, mA and time. During fluoroscopy a warning light will show on the console, indicating radiation is being emitted from the X-ray tube. A buzzer sounds after a set time limit, approximately five minutes, to indicate the duration of fluoroscopy which can be reset so that screening can continue.

IMAGE INTENSIFIER SYSTEM

The system consists of an image intensifier, a television camera and a television monitor. The television camera is connected directly to the television monitor and forms a closed circuit, unlike conventional broadcast television which uses radio waves.

The image intensifer converts the X-ray pattern it receives into a corresponding light image. This is changed into an electrical signal by the television camera so that it can be seen on the television monitor.

Image intensifier

The image intensifier (see Figure 5.7) consists of an evacuated glass tube, but with more modern units it is of all-metal construction. It contains an input screen (phosphor) and photo cathode, focusing electrodes, anode and output screen (phosphor).[15,16]

The tube, except for the input screen, is surrounded by a light-tight, anti-magnetic, protective metal casing which has a lead equivalent of 2 mm if used at 100 kV, and plus 0.01 mm lead equivalent for each extra kV from 100 to 150 kV.[17] The front covering of the intensifier is usually made of titanium foil. It must absorb little of the primary radiation which has passed through the patient, to allow the radiation to reach the input screen.

Input screen

This can be from 12.5 to 35 cm in diameter. The 35 cm screen has only become available recently, so most older simulators have a smaller input screen of 22–25 cm, which is a slight disadvantage when trying to image large areas. The input screen can be flat or curved; a flat screen will produce a better image because the edges of the image will be less blurred.

The screen is coated with a phosphor, which is a fluorescent material (see Chapter 2), such as caesium iodide. When X-rays reach this material

Figure 5.7: Diagram of an image intensifier. With acknowledgement to *X-Ray Equipment for Student Radiographers* (Chesney and Chesney, 3rd edn, Blackwell Scientific Publications Ltd).

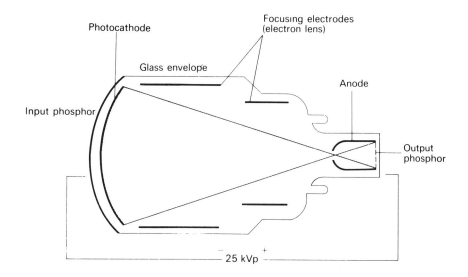

they are converted into light photons which then fall on the photocathode behind the input screen. As the photocathode receives light it will emit electrons in proportion to the intensity of the light it receives. The input screen and photocathode must be in very close proximity or the image which is received will lose detail.

Focusing electrodes (electron lens)

This is a series of positively charged electrodes which are plated onto the inside surface of the glass envelope. The focusing lens causes the image to be inverted, as it focuses the electrons to a specific point on the opposite side of the output phosphor (see Figure 5.7). The focusing of the electron beam is necessary to ensure good definition of the image.

Accelerating anode

The anode is near the output end of the image intensifier. There is a voltage difference of 25 kV between the photocathode and anode so that the electrons emitted from the photocathode are pulled across the tube towards the anode and the output screen.

Output screen

This is a fluorescent screen and is coated with a phosphor, commonly zinc cadmium sulphide activated by silver. It is 1.25–3.5 cm in size. When the electrons from the photocathode strike the output screen, because they have been accelerated, they produce more light photons than were present from the input screen. The light photons are emitted in the same pattern as the original from the input screen but greatly reduced in size. These two factors, the gain of light photons and the minification of the image, cause the image at the output screen to be brighter than at the input screen.

A thin layer of aluminium is plated onto the output screen to prevent light photons passing back to the photocathode and producing more electrons which are not part of the original image.

The output screen of the intensifier is in close contact with a lens system which will convert the inverted image to the usual orientation; the image is then transferred to the television camera. In more modern intensifiers a fibre optic coupling is used to transfer the image, which consists of a plano-concave fibre optic disc and is linked directly with the television camera. This will increase the light transmission, reduce scatter and the image distortion.[17]

The advantage of the image intensifier is that it can convert a weak initial image into a much brighter one. This means only a small amount of incident radiation is needed to produce a useful image. (For exposure factors when using the image intensifier see Chapter 6.)

IMAGE SCANNING SYSTEM

The image scanning system consists of television camera and camera control unit used in a closed circuit with a television monitor. The image from the output screen of the intensifier is focused onto the target assembly of the television camera, which is converted into an electronic (video) signal that can be reassembled and viewed on the television monitor.

Television camera

The vidicon television camera is generally used with most types of simulators.[17,18] The most important part is the vidicon tube.

Vidicon tube

This is a small evacuated tube 15 cm in length and 2.5 cm in diameter which is surrounded by focusing and deflecting coils. The tube has at one end a glass face-plate in front of the signal electrode and photoconductive layer (target), with the accelerating cylinder (anode) along the tube, and at the other end a cathode with an electron gun (see Figure 5.8).

Glass face-plate

This maintains the vacuum in the tube.

Signal electrode

This is an electrical conductor with a positive potential of 25 V. The signal

Figure 5.8: Vidicon camera tube. With acknowledgement to *X-Ray Equipment for Student Radiographers* (Chesney and Chesney, 3rd edn, Blackwell Scientific Publications Ltd).

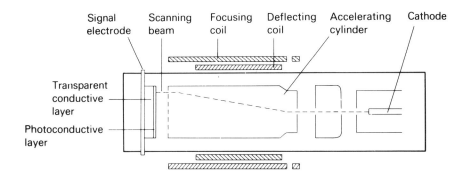

electrode transmits the electronic signal to the television monitor to allow the image to be viewed. The conductive transparent layer, which is made of zinc oxide, is part of the signal electrode. This allows the light photons from the image intensifier to reach the target.

Photoconductive layer (target)

This contains a thin film of material, antimony trisulphide, which is a photoconductor and will emit electrons when exposed to light. This material is in the form of tiny globules within a mica matrix. When the globules absorb the light photons, emitted from the output screen of the intensifier, they emit electrons. These are attracted to the signal electrode and removed from the tube. This flow of electrons is not recorded; it is a clipped signal. The globules, having lost electrons, become positively charged and form an electrical image, an exact replica of the original from the input screen of the image intensifier. This charge is eventually turned into the electronic signal which helps to form the television image.

Accelerating cylinder (anode)

The anode extends along the tube as a fine wire mesh towards the target and has a positive potential of 250–300 V.

Cathode

This is at the opposite end of the vidicon to the target, and contains an electron gun, which produces electrons by thermionic emission. The electron beam from the cathode scans the electrical image which is stored in the mica matrix of the target.

Initially the electrons from the cathode are accelerated towards the anode because of the positive potential of the anode, and then are decelerated before they reach the target to help straighten their path so they strike the target perpendicularly. The wire mesh of the anode and signal electrode form the decelerating field. There are focusing and deflecting coils around the tube to ensure the electron beam is brought to a point (as it scans a dot picture) and is moved up and down to the left and right for scanning purposes.[19]

Scanning

This is like reading a book: the electron beam from the cathode scans the target from left to right, in straight lines, and when it reaches the bottom of the target it rapidly flies back to start at the top left, and then continues scanning left to right, and so on.[18]

The vidicon camera uses a double-interlacing system, which means the frame, which is made up of 625 lines, is scanned twice. First the odd lines are scanned (312.5 lines per scan) and then the even lines are scanned (again 312.5 lines per scan) to complete the whole frame (see Figure 5.9).

Figure 5.9: Interlaced scanning. The odd-numbered lines are scanned first (striped areas), followed by the even lines (clear areas). With acknowledgement to *X-Ray Equipment for Student Radiographers* (Chesney and Chesney, 3rd edn, Blackwell Scientific Publications Ltd).

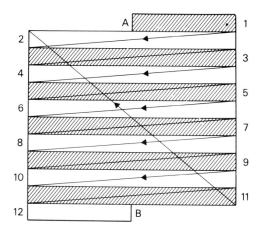

As the electron beam scans the target it discharges the positively charged globules and a current flows through the conductive signal electrode of the vidicon; this current forms the electronic signal. Not all the globules are discharged at the same time — only a small cluster, a dot, each instant. Therefore a series of electronic pulses, each corresponding to an exact area on the target, is reassembled into a visible image by the television monitor.

Camera control unit

This contains the power supply and all the controls which regulate the camera. It also amplifies the electronic signal and synchronises the signal between the camera and the television monitor.

TELEVISION MONITOR

The television monitor consists of an evacuated glass tube which is a cathode ray tube.[18] It has a large front surface which is coated with a luminescent material and at the opposite end is the electron gun, grid and the anode (see Figure 5.10). The electron gun produces a beam of electrons which is controlled by the grid.

Grid

This uses the electronic signal from the television camera to regulate the number of electrons in the beam which will reach the front screen. A bright

Figure 5.10: Diagram of a cathode ray tube. (Reproduced by permission of E. Forster and MTP Press Ltd.)

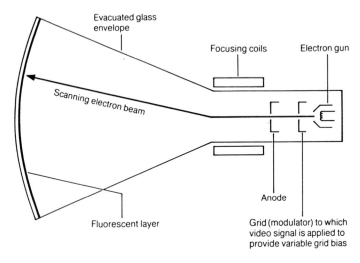

area will show on the television monitor when a large number of electrons are allowed to reach the opposite end of the cathode ray tube, and a dark area when the electron flow is almost completely cut off.

This beam of electrons is then accelerated towards the anode because of the positive potential on the anode of about 10 kV. The electrons are focused by the focusing coils and the deflection coils cause the electrons to scan the large front surface of the cathode ray tube. The electron beam scans in the same manner as the vidicon, and is synchronised with the vidicon. When the electrons hit the front screen they fluoresce and light photons are produced, in the original pattern as emitted from the intensifier, and the image can be viewed on the television monitor.

This image is in the form of dots which produce a pattern in horizontal lines, called scan lines, as already mentioned. There are 625 lines per frame and each horizontal line has approximately 300 pieces of information, which produces an image with good definition.

The television monitor contains controls for regulating brightness and contrast to help improve the image received from the television camera, which unfortunately becomes degraded as it passes through the television system.

Cost

The image intensifier system, including the television camera and monitor, can cost from £35,000 to £45,000 (1986/7 prices).

Video tape recording

Some radiotherapy departments have a system where magnetic (video) tape cassettes are used to record images for localisation with the simulator (see Chapter 6), instead of the usual film screen combinations (see Chapters 1 and 2). The image intensifier system produces the images and the electronic signal from the vidicon is stored on magnetic tape.

The video tape is a plastic tape coated with ferrous oxide. It is passed in front of an electromagnet, the recording head, which is fed with the electronic signal from the vidicon and magnetises the tape in proportion to the strength and frequency of the signal. To play back, the tape is passed in front of a replay head, which induces a similar signal from the tape to the replay head, so that the images can then be viewed on a television monitor.[19]

Image storage tube

With the help of a computer the television monitor is able to store images which can be recalled on the monitor screen by switching, and then return to normal dynamic viewing. In other words, an image can be viewed at leisure via the image intensifier system without giving the patient more exposure.[18] This is useful when using the simulator for fluoroscopy (see Chapter 6).

MECHANICAL SYSTEM

The movements of the simulator should match as far as possible the same movements and accuracy in positioning as the treatment units. There is a need for care with mechanical tolerances of the simulator (see below) which require specialised engineering and make the equipment expensive. Most manufacturers now sell the simulator with both the mechanical system and the X-ray system together, and this costs from £210,000 to £240,000 (1986/7 prices).

Gantry and stand

The gantry and stand (see Figure 5.11) support at the upper end the collimator assembly, X-ray tube and housing, and at the lower end the image intensifier and television camera. The gantry must be rigid and isocentrically mounted to be able to rotate in the same manner as on the treatment units.

The isocentre

This is defined as the same centre for rotation, and means that the gantry,

119

Figure 5.11: Diagram of the simulator. (Courtesy of Philips Medical Systems.)
A = Gantry
B = Stand
C = Collimator system
D = Image intensifier

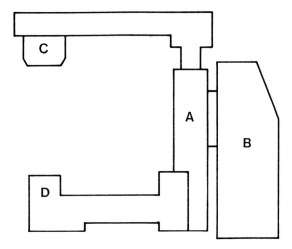

collimator and couch will rotate about the same specified point.[20] The rotation about the isocentre must be within an accuracy of ±2 mm, the usual practical accepted tolerance as for the treatment units.

FAD

The distance from the focus of the X-ray tube to the isocentre is called the focus to axis distance (FAD). It can be varied in most simulators generally within a range of 80–140 cm. The FAD is usually changed by raising or lowering the collimator assembly.

SSD

When using the simulator it is common practice to refer to the SSD rather than the FAD. The SSD is the distance from the skin of the patient to the source or focus of the X-ray tube. It is usually indicated by a scale (optical range-finder) which is projected onto the patient's skin, and when the SSD is set at the isocentre this relates to the FAD.

Collimator system

The collimator system at the upper end of the gantry contains the X-ray collimator assembly, field defining wires, field illumination assembly and scale for collimator rotation (see Figure 5.12).

Figure 5.12: Diagram of the collimator system. (Courtesy of Philips Medical Systems.)

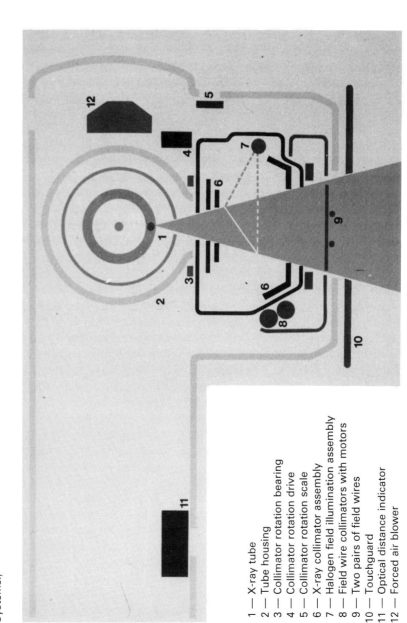

1 — X-ray tube
2 — Tube housing
3 — Collimator rotation bearing
4 — Collimator rotation drive
5 — Collimator rotation scale
6 — X-ray collimator assembly
7 — Halogen field illumination assembly
8 — Field wire collimators with motors
9 — Two pairs of field wires
10 — Touchguard
11 — Optical distance indicator
12 — Forced air blower

Collimator assembly

This consists of four motorised lead blades. These outer collimator blades move from 0 × 0 cm to 50 × 50 cm, and can move independently of each other. The actual treatment field is delineated by a set of field defining wires and the outer collimator blades allow an adjacent area to be seen on the image. This system helps with location and protection of vital structures close to the treatment area (see Figure 5.13).

Field defining wires

These are two pairs of wires, 0.5 mm in diameter, which can be moved to show rectangular field sizes from 3 × 3 cm to 45 × 45 cm. In some newer units these wires can move independently. The field defining wires indicate the treatment field size, for the set FAD, and the read-out should be regularly checked for accuracy. Most units have a central cross-wire in the middle of the field defining wires.

Field illumination assembly

An optical system projects a light beam which indicates the position of the lead collimators and field defining wires. It is important that the X-ray beam and the area delineated by the field defining wires are accurately aligned for the images produced to be of relevance. This should be checked when the simulator is installed, and at regular intervals.[21]

Figure 5.13: Field area defined and adjacent area by collimator blades. (Courtesy of Philips Medical Systems.)

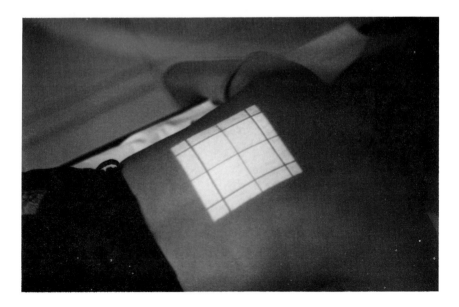

Collimator rotation

The collimator can rotate around the centre of the field in the same plane. The degree of rotation is shown on the scale around the outside of the collimator. The collimator rotation must be accurate with reference to the centre of the field defining wires, and to try to ensure that a motorised collimator system is used.

Image intensifier assembly

At the lower end of the gantry is the image intensifier assembly (see Figure 5.11). It can be moved in various directions — laterally, longitudinally and vertically. Care has to be taken when moving the intensifier as it is quite bulky so that it does not collide with the couch. With most modern simulators there is an anti-collision mechanism or a touchguard to help prevent damaging equipment, and with new technology the size of the intensifier is being reduced. In some units the intensifier has automatic centring, and it will automatically move to coincide with the central axis of the radiation beam and then stop at this point.

The top surface of the intensifier usually has a support or carriage to hold a cassette (35 × 43 cm) and a secondary radiation grid (see Chapter 2), which is placed in front of the cassette. The Varian Ximatron CX simulator has the facility for accepting an ionisation chamber system for automatic exposure control. This is placed between the grid and cassette, and automatically causes the exposure to terminate when the correct amount of radiation has reached the film to give the desired density.[22]

Couch

The couch for the simulator should be identical to the couches used for the treatment units in the department, usually flat-topped and hard. It must be isocentrically mounted so it rotates about the isocentre and its vertical movements go through the isocentre. The couch should also be able to move laterally and longitudinally.[23]

There must be removable panels similar to those on the treatment couches, allowing either a centrespine or a side rail system. The modern designs are made from carbon fibre generally with a size of 240 cm length × 50 cm width, and able to take a weight distribution of about 130 kg over the isocentre with no distortion.

The couch must be radiolucent so that the images produced, with an X-ray film in a cassette under the couch and by using the image intensifier system, are not degraded.

Local and remote control

The movements of the gantry, collimator blades, field defining wires, rotation of the collimator, couch and intensifier have a mechanism for remote and local control. The exception is the rotation of the couch, which is usually local control only to help prevent collisions with the rest of the equipment.[23]

Pedestal or ceiling-suspended units are used for local control with digital or mechanical scale showing the parameters set, and with some simulators this information is seen by using television monitors. The equipment for local control is in the same area as the simulator, whereas the console for remote control is adjacent to the simulator within a protected area or completely separate room (see Figure 5.14).

The Varian CX Ximatron has an auto-set-up control which allows the various parameters to be pre-set on the remote console and will then automatically move the equipment. This gives a fast 'set-up' procedure, and to ensure safety there must be anti-collision bars on the equipment and the orientation of the equipment should be controlled by computer.

Computer compatibility

The simulator should be designed for computer compatibility with the treatment planning computer and the computer system on the treatment units.[23] This will enable data from the simulator to be sent directly to the treatment planning computer and back to the simulator. It will also allow the parameters from the simulator to be sent to the treatment units which have the record and verification system.[24]

Accessories

As well as the main equipment described above the simulator generally has accessory equipment to help with the localisation and verification of treatment fields (see Chapter 6).

Shielding tray facility

Most simulators are able to attach a device to simulate the shielding tray.[23] This is used to hold lead blocks which are placed in the path of the radiation to protect areas not requiring any treatment. The shielding tray facility is at the same distance from the focus of the radiation as on the treatment unit. It enables positioning of shielding blocks to verify treatment areas (see Figure 5.15). This is a more effective way of checking the shielding than using the conventional lead solder wire on the surface of the patient, to define the shielding area.

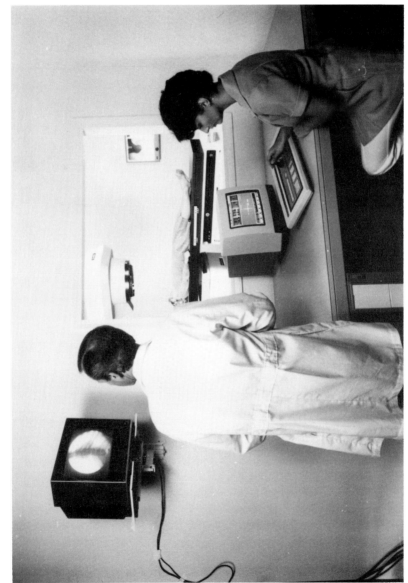

Figure 5.14: Simulator and remote control area. (Courtesy of Varian.)

Figure 5.15: Simulator with shielding tray attachment. (Courtesy of Varian.)

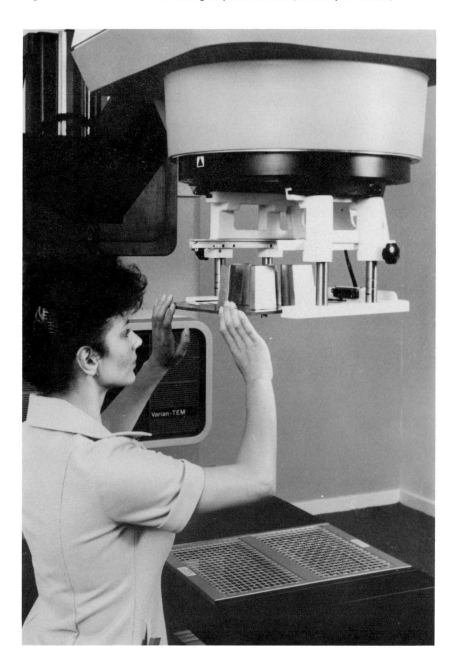

Figure 5.16: Electron treatment simulation. (Courtesy of Varian.)

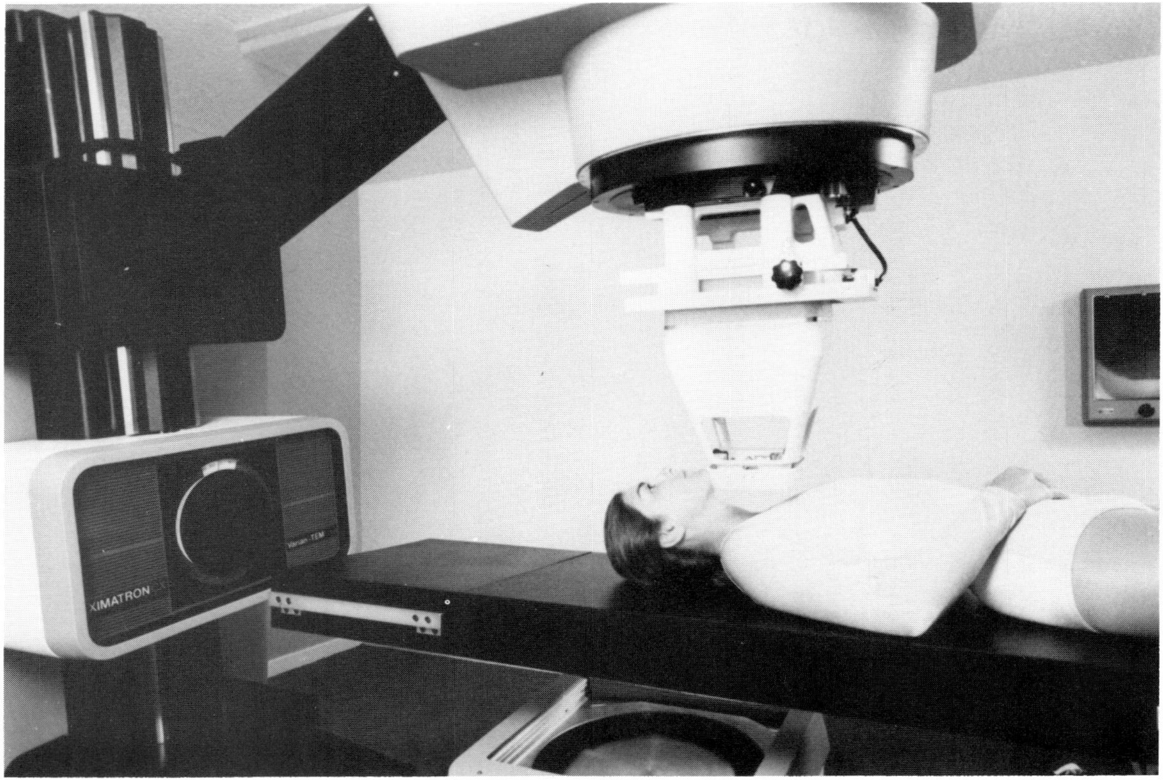

Electron treatment simulation

The Varian Ximatron CX simulator has an accessory mount which accepts actual electron applicators (see Figure 5.16). Treatment with electrons[25] is usually carried out on the linear accelerator treatment unit using very bulky applicators. It is useful to spend time positioning the simulated applicators for any difficult areas, which occur quite often with electron treatment 'set-ups'.

Setting-up aids

Lasers or axis lights are used to help position the patient so that a reproducible 'set-up' can be achieved (see Chapter 6).

Lasers

Low-power lasers are used as an aid to positioning the patient on the simulator.[23] They are quite safe but the only caution the manufacturers suggest is that the laser beam is not stared at directly. There are usually two horizontal lasers: one transverse laser and a sagittal laser. Where the lasers meet is the isocentre, and it is necessary to check this regularly. The sagittal laser can be used to define the mid-line of the patient as it projects longitudinally down the couch, and is in line with the centre of the delineated field area.

Axis lights

These are also used to define the isocentre and usually consist of three lights, two horizontal, and one vertical. They are in line with the central axis of the beam and the vertical axis light is only seen when the gantry is angled away from 0°. Unlike the lasers they do not show a long continuous line, but are in the form of a small cross. It is important that they should be checked regularly to ensure they align at the isocentre.

Built-in contouring devices

To complete localising procedures it is necessary to obtain an outline of the patient, usually around the central plane of the defined area (see Chapter 6). The contour should be a true representation and an accurate record.

One system used is like a pantograph, and consists of a wall-mounted frame and tracing hook with a pen on the free end.[23] It is coordinated so that as the hook is gently moved across the relevant outline the pen automatically draws the shape on the board and paper situated overhead. Another method is to use computed tomography or transverse analogue tomography (see Chapter 7). It is also possible to produce the outline using ultrasound (see Chapter 8).

ROUTINE CARE OF EQUIPMENT

The simulator is a very expensive and sensitive piece of equipment. It should be treated with respect as it has to comply with a high degree of accuracy. Most tolerance limits are between ±2 mm, so any bad handling could render the equipment outside the tolerance limits. Care must be taken with all mechanical movements, especially when using remote control, as not all parts of the equipment are always in view.

Regular servicing of the simulator is important and any mechanical or electrical faults should be recorded. The manufacturers usually suggest a 3- or 6-month service contract. (For more details on quality assurance (acceptance tests and quality control) of the simulator see Reference 21 and Further Reading.)

DESIGN OF THE ROOM

The simulator requires a room which contains the simulator frame with X-ray tube and intensifier, couch and local control equipment. An adjacent or completely separate control room is needed for the generator console, remote control equipment, television monitor and viewing area.[26]

Adequate room for housing the simulator frame should be about 6 m square to allow for isocentric gantry movements through 180° with the various accessory attachments. The entry to the simulator should be large enough for a bed or trolley to be wheeled into the room.

The room must be shielded to reduce the radiation hazard (see below) and have adequate ventilation and variable light control. It is important to have sound-proofing between the simulator room and the adjacent control room as it is quite often used for teaching purposes. However, there must be communication between the two areas by a microphone or intercom.

A large panoramic lead glass window or thick plate glass 0.5 × 1 m in size is desirable between the simulator and control room. The window should be parallel to the long axis of the couch to get a good view of the patient, and so that the patient can also see the staff more easily. The height of the window should allow the operator in the control room to see the patient and the simulator equipment comfortably. The blind side of the couch should be viewed by use of a mirror or television camera and monitor. It should be possible to draw a curtain or screen over the window for privacy — for instance, when the medical staff are examining the patient.

The control area should have variable lighting to ensure adequate viewing conditions of the image on the television screen or on the viewing box, and good ventilation. A minimum area of 6 × 4 m is recommended, with easy access to an automatic processor and darkroom if necessary (see Chapter 4).

RADIATION PROTECTION

It is necessary that the simulator room is reinforced with a high atomic number, and high density material, which will attenuate ionising radiation, in accordance with the 1985 Ionising Radiations Regulations.[27] This is so that patients and staff in rooms adjacent to the simulator are protected against the radiation hazard. A primary barrier is required to shield the primary radiation, and secondary barriers to shield secondary radiation or scatter.[28]

Primary barrier

This is the lead lining of the X-ray tube housing which attenuates all the radiation produced from the focal spot except that which goes through the translucent window as the useful beam. Extra protection may be needed for doors, ceiling and walls if they are in the path of the primary beam.

Secondary barrier

This is needed for the remote control area as it should not be in the path of the primary beam.

Lead, which has high atomic number and density, is one of the most effective attenuators of radiation at the low energies (50–150 kV) which are used with the simulator. Other materials, such as barium plaster or lead plywood, used for protection, are quoted as a lead equivalent. This is the thickness of lead in millimetres which gives the same protection as the barrier.

Care when imaging to patients and staff

Patients

Although the patient is probably going to receive a high dose of radiation in the area for treatment, it is important when using the simulator to take care with adjacent vital structures, such as the lens of the eye and reproductive organs, especially in young patients. Adequate shielding should be used, shielding blocks in the beam, lead aprons to cover the patient or gonad protection. This accessory equipment should be checked periodically to see it adequately attenuates the radiation.

To help reduce the radiation it is good practice to close down the collimators so that only the vital anatomy is imaged. This will also improve the definition of the image as it reduces scatter. When screening large field areas, as the image intensifier screen will not always cover the whole area, care should be taken to stop screening when the intensifier is moving from the upper to the lower border, if the area in between is not of interest. This will prevent unnecessary radiation being given to the patient.

Staff

It is important that the local rules and/or a scheme of work, for the simulator area, is displayed and brought to the attention of all staff.[27] It is usual practice for staff to be in the control room when irradiating the patient, as no one other than the patient should be in the useful beam.[27] An automatic signal indicator should show on the control panel when the X-ray tube is energised or the intensifier is being used. At the same time a warning signal should show at any entrance to the simulator room. All the controls which cause the production of X-rays should be clearly labelled, and there should be an effective means of terminating the exposure quickly and isolating the equipment from the mains.[27]

REFERENCES

1. Forster, E. (1985) *Equipment for Diagnostic Radiography*, MTP Press, Lancaster, pp. 56-9.
2. Chesney, D.N. and Chesney, M.O. (1984) *X-Ray Equipment for Student Radiographers*, 3rd edn, Blackwell Scientific Publications, Oxford, pp. 237-49.
3. McCullough, E.C. and Earle, J.D. (1979) 'The selection, acceptance, testing and quality control of radiotherapy treatment simulators', *Radiology*, **131**, 226.
4. Wilks, R. (1981) *Principles of Radiological Physics*, Churchill Livingstone, Edinburgh, pp. 88-93.
5. Forster, E. (1985) *Equipment for Diagnostic Radiography*, MTP Press, Lancaster, pp. 63-8.
6. Wilks, R. (1981) *Principles of Radiological Physics*, Churchill Livingstone, Edinburgh, pp. 285-6.
7. Forster, E. (1985) *Equipment for Diagnostic Radiography*, MTP Press, Lancaster, pp. 62-5.
8. Chesney, D.N. and Chesney, M.O. (1984) *X-Ray Equipment*, 3rd edn, Blackwell Scientific Publications, Oxford, pp. 249-57, 257-61.
9. Forster, E. (1985) *Equipment for Radiography*, MTP Press, Lancaster, pp. 78-9.
10. Chesney, D.N. and Chesney, M.O. (1984) *X-Ray Equipment*, 3rd edn, Blackwell Scientific Publications, Oxford, pp. 29-85.
11. Forster, E. (1985) *Equipment for Radiography*, MTP Press, Lancaster, pp. 11-43, 54.
12. Wilks, R. (1981) *Principles of Radiological Physics*, Churchill Livingstone, Edinburgh, pp. 181-200, 272-5.
13. Chesney, D.N. and Chesney, M.O. (1984) *X-Ray Equipment*, 3rd edn, Blackwell Scientific Publications, Oxford, pp. 1-25, 89-91.
14. Bomford, C.K., Craig, L.M., Hanna, F.A., *et al.* (1981) 'Treatment simulators', *British Journal of Radiology*, Supplement 16, p. 25.
15. Curry, T.S., Dowdey, J.E. and Murray Jr, C. (1984) *Christensen's Introduction to the Physics of Diagnostic Radiology*, 3rd edn, Lea and Febiger, Philadelphia, pp. 190-9.
16. Chesney, D.N. and Chesney, M.O. (1984) *X-Ray Equipment*, 3rd edn, Blackwell Scientific Publications, Oxford, pp. 383-9.

17. Forster, E. (1985) *Equipment for Radiography*, MTP Press, Lancaster, pp. 105-8, 109-11.
18. Chesney, D.N. and Chesney, M.O. (1984) *X-Ray Equipment*, 3rd edn, Blackwell Scientific Publications, Oxford, pp. 372-83, 402.
19. Curry, T.S., Dowdey, J.E. and Murray Jr, R.C. (1984) *Christensen's Introduction to the Physics of Diagnostic Radiology*, 3rd edn, Lea and Febiger, Philadelphia, pp. 230-2, 238-42.
20. Bleehen, N.M., Glatstein, E. and Haybittle, J.L. (1983) *Radiation Therapy Planning*, Marcel Dekker, New York, pp. 113-14.
21. McCullough, E.C. and Earle, J.D. (1979) 'The selection, acceptance, testing and quality control of treatment simulators', *Radiology*, **131**, pp. 227-29.
22. Forster, E. (1985) *Equipment for Radiography*, MTP Press, Lancaster, p. 46.
23. Bomford, C.K., Craig, L.M., Hanna, F.A., *et al.* (1981) 'Treatment simulators', *British Journal of Radiology*, Supplement 16, pp. 9-13.
24. Bleehen, N.M., Glatstein, E. and Haybittle, J.L. (1983) *Radiation Therapy Planning*, Marcel Dekker, New York, pp. 300-80.
25. Bleehen, N.M., Glatstein, E. and Haybittle, J.L. (1983) *Radiation Therapy Planning*, Marcel Dekker, New York, pp. 343-92.
26. Bomford, C.K., Craig, L.M., Hanna, F.A., *et al.* (1981) 'Treatment simulators', *British Journal of Radiology*, Supplement 16, pp. 14-16.
27. Health and Safety Commission (1985) *The Ionising Radiations Regulations*, Her Majesty's Stationery Office, Part 1, pp. 3, 26, 185; Part 2, pp. 27-8.
28. Meredith, W.J. and Massey, J.B. (1977) *Fundamental Physics of Radiology*, 3rd edn, Wright, Bristol, pp. 638-48.

Private communications

O. Deaville; M. McClellan; J. Stock.

Manufacturers' literature

Agfa Gevaert, 'T.V. Monitor, Monitor Photography, Vidicon'.
Philips Medical Systems, 'Localiser/Simulator'.
Picker International, 'X-Ray Tubes PX'.
Varian, 'Ximatron CX Radiotherapy Simulators', Equipment Specifications.
Varian C Series Radiotherapy Simulators.

FURTHER READING

Przeslak, A.J. (1987) 'Quality assurance in simulators', *Radiography*, **53**(607), 27-30.

6

The Use of the Simulator (including procedures with radiological contrast media)

The simulator is used to produce images in the form of a radiograph (see Figure 6.1), xeroradiograph (see Chapter 1) or during fluoroscopy (screening) to localise and verify treatment field areas for radiotherapy.

LOCALISATION

The aim is to correctly identify the area for treatment by using the above imaging techniques (producing a radiograph and fluoroscopy will be explained later in this chapter). The localisation procedure can be complicated or very simple, depending on whether it is a radical or palliative treatment.

Radical treatment

This involves a treatment which is aimed at curing the patient. Great care and precision should be taken with localisation to ensure an accurate, reproducible 'set-up' for treatment. The radical treatment usually requires a treatment plan.

Treatment plan

So that the target volume, an area which includes a margin around the tumour, receives a well-defined dose of radiation, a treatment plan is produced.

The treatment plan requires a cross-sectional outline through the centre of the target volume. This usually shows a transverse contour around the surface of the patient, with the target volume and any vital structures close to the area being treated drawn onto the diagram.[1-3] Various radiation fields are placed on the outline to give the best method of treating the target volume, with as small an amount of radiation as possible going to normal tissue.

Figure 6.1: Radiograph — anteroposterior (AP) pelvis. (Courtesy of the Middlesex Hospital Radiotherapy Department.)

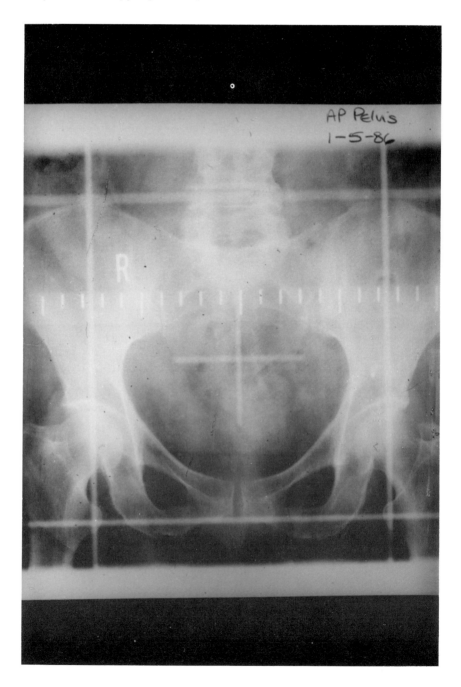

This dosimetry is worked out either by manual planning or computer planning.[4,5] The computer method is much quicker than manual planning, and modern systems are able to be linked directly to the simulator, the treatment units and with the CT scanner (see Chapter 7).

Positioning of the patient

The first step to producing accurate images for treatment purposes is to position the patient correctly.[6,7] It is important to use the lasers (see Chapter 5) to help align the patient in the longitudinal and horizontal planes. The approximate centre of the treatment field should then be positioned to the centre of the optical field delineated by the wires and collimators (see Chapter 5), with the correct treating distance for the treatment unit to be used. The next step is to screen the area to define exactly the centre or borders of the area for treatment.

Fluoroscopy (screening)

The image intensifier produces images which can be viewed on a television monitor in an adjacent area to the simulator (see Chapter 5). It is placed perpendicular to the source of radiation and is generally under or lateral to the couch.

Exposure factors for screening

These can be preset or adjusted manually. The kV can usually be set from 70 kVp to 120 kVp and the screening current varies from 2 to 5 mA (see General guide to exposure factors, later in this chapter).

For a good image to be produced it is useful to get the intensifier as close as possible to the area being screened, and as the intensifier equipment is quite bulky care has to be taken when moving either the couch, gantry or intensifier. It is important to try to reduce secondary scatter which will degrade the image (see Chapter 2). This is achieved by closing down the collimator blades (see Chapter 5) as far as possible while still showing the necessary information; it also helps to use a secondary radiation grid (see Chapter 2).

During fluoroscopy the intensifier is used to check the borders of the treatment field. The images are viewed instantaneously on a television monitor and if corrections have to be made to any parameters, for instance the width, length or borders, this can be done by moving either the field defining wires or the couch by remote control (see Chapter 5). If the field area is too large to be completely seen on the monitor each border and surrounding area can be screened, but it is not usually necessary to screen the entire length or width of the area, as this only gives more radiation to the patient.

When screening the timer will sound after five minutes, and can then be reset; but it is a reminder of the amount of time the patient is receiving radiation. Care should be taken when screening (for more details see Chapter 5). It is useful to be able to use an image store when using fluoroscopy (see Chapter 5). The images of interest can be stored on the monitor and viewed at leisure without continually irradiating the patient.

The radiograph

Orthogonal radiographs (films taken at 90° to each other) are then produced of the area to be treated.

Duplitised film (see Chapter 1) in a cassette containing intensifying screens (see Chapter 2) is generally used, which can be kept as a permanent copy. It is also possible to use xeroradiography for this procedure (more details can be found in Chapter 1). The projections of the radiographs are usually an anteroposterior (AP) radiograph (see Figure 6.1) which localises structures in the coronal plane, and a lateral radiograph (see Figure 6.2) to locate the target area with respect to the anterior surface of the patient and adjacent structures (sagittal plane).

Positioning the cassette

This should be placed perpendicularly to the source of radiation to prevent distortion of the image.[8] It is better to have the cassette as close to the specific area of the patient as possible, as this reduces magnification. It also gives less penumbra and therefore reduced geometric unsharpness of the image (see Chapter 3).

Magnification

As the X-ray beam diverges the image produced on the film is always slightly larger than the original image, and this effect is called magnification. It depends on the distance between the patient and the film, and the distance between the patient and the focus of the X-rays. The minimum amount of magnification is produced if the film is close to the patient and the patient is at a long distance from the focus of the X-ray tube.[8]

The magnification can be measured, which is useful in order to calculate the image size on the film relative to the size on the actual patient (see Figure 6.3).

Magnification rulers

These are used to work out the average magnification factor for the radiograph. The rulers have metal strips at centimetre intervals and are placed

Figure 6.2: Radiograph — lateral pelvis; double-exposure technique. Collimators closed down, then opened out to allow the anterior surface to be seen.

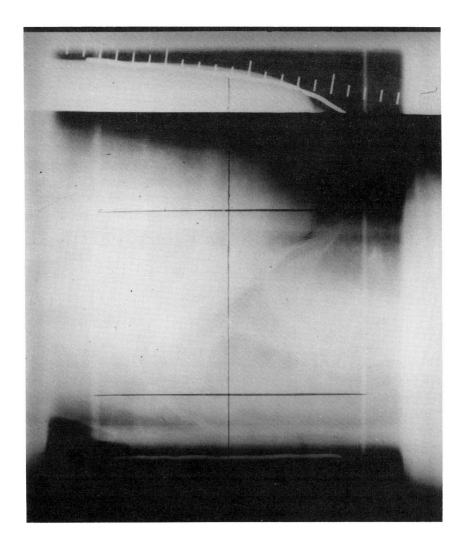

on the patient at the centre of the treatment field. When the image is viewed it will show the interval between the metal strips has been increased, and the ratio between these two measurements will be the magnification factor.

When producing a radiograph it is important to use radio-opaque markers in the form of lead letters (see Figure 6.1). These are usually placed on the patient and will identify certain features of the image such as right or left and if the patient is prone or supine.

137

Figure 6.3: Diagram used to calculate the degree of magnification of the original object. (Reproduced by permission of Kodak Ltd.)

$$M = \frac{a+b}{a}$$

M = magnification factor
a = distance from focus to object
b = distance from object to film

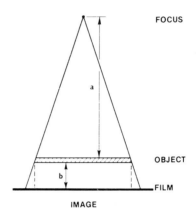

IMAGE

The exposure

To produce the radiograph an exposure is needed which consists of kV, mA and time or mAs, which are set on the generator control console (see Chapter 5). To ensure sharp images and sharp field defining wires on the image it is important to try to use the fine focus rather than broad focus; however, this will depend on the rating of the X-ray tube (see Chapter 5).

General guide to exposure factors

The exposure factors will vary depending on the type of generator, the focal spot of the X-ray tube (see Chapter 5), the film screen combination and whether a secondary radiation grid is used (see Chapter 2). The following is a rough guide to exposure factors.

The kV

This influences the contrast of the image and the quality of the radiation. A low kV (60 kV) results in a high-contrast image which predominantly shows bony detail, and soft tissue will not be so easily identified. A high kV (120 kV) image will demonstrate bone and soft tissue with low contrast. This is useful for localising the chest if it is necessary to see the structures of

138

the mediastinum more clearly than the ribs. At high kV it is important to use a secondary radiation grid, whereas below 70 kV this is not necessary (see Chapter 2). For large patients higher kV (above 75 kV) is needed so that the X-rays will penetrate the area being imaged.

The mAs

The quantity of radiation required, which is the mAs, depends on the thickness and density of the area. A low mAs (16 mAs) is required to image the chest as it is mainly air and does not greatly attenuate the radiation. For a lateral pelvic radiograph, as the distance through the patient is usually large and this area contains dense structures, a high mAs (200 mAs) is needed.

Time

If the time can be set separately from the mA then the shortest possible time will give a less blurred image as there will be less involuntary movement. However, this will depend on the rating of the tube (see Chapter 5).

Distance

The focus to film distance influences the density of the radiograph because of the inverse square law.[9] A greater quantity of radiation is needed for a useful image if the cassette is at a long distance from the source of radiation. The positioning of the cassette relative to the patient, and the distance from the patient to the focus, will also affect the geometric unsharpness (see Chapter 3) and magnification of the radiograph, as already explained in this chapter.

Acceptability of the radiograph

A few simple checks should be made to see that the required information for the procedure has been shown on the radiograph:

  Identification of patient and date
  Inclusion of required anatomy
  Field defining markers
  Radio-opaque marker(s) correctly positioned
  Magnification ruler(s) correctly positioned
  Gantry angle
  Collimation and required density and contrast on the image
  Absence of unsharpness and artefacts

When the area for treatment is satisfactorily located it is important to mark the centre and/or borders of the treatment field on the patient as a tiny indelible tattoo, or on the immobilisation shell. This is a clear plastic shell used mostly for head and neck treatments 'tailor-made' to fit each patient to prevent movement during treatment.[10]

The AP and lateral radiographs from the simulator are used in conjunction with other investigations such as diagnostic radiographs, computed tomography (CT scans), ultrasound scans and magnetic resonance imaging (MRI scans) to mark the target volume on the cross-sectional outline. This will then be used for planning the area for treatment (see earlier in this chapter). (For more information about localising techniques see Bleehen *et al.*, Bentel *et al.*, and Dobbs and Barrett, Further Reading.)

Palliative treatment

This kind of treatment is important for alleviating pain and generally reducing distressing symptoms. It is still necessary to pinpoint the area to be treated as accurately as possible, but the actual treatment techniques are less complicated and there is usually no treatment plan. For localisation purposes the area for treatment can be screened and usually only one radiograph produced (see Figure 6.4).

VERIFICATION

When the treatment area has been localised it is important that the final treatment 'set-up' is checked. This can be done by using the simulator or with the treatment unit as described in Chapter 1.

Radical treatment

The patient is correctly aligned, and then the simulator is positioned according to the treatment plan. Images are produced to check that the specified areas of the treatment are correct. It is quite often necessary to image oblique views as the angles for the treatment fields are not always at 0°, 90°, 180° or 270°, and it is sometimes difficult to distinguish structures on these images. Moving the simulator in this way will also help to check if the fields can be achieved practically on the treatment unit.

Palliative treatments

These field areas are not usually verified on a separate occasion, as this is usually combined with the localisation procedure. However, it may be

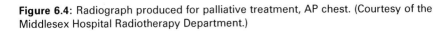

Figure 6.4: Radiograph produced for palliative treatment, AP chest. (Courtesy of the Middlesex Hospital Radiotherapy Department.)

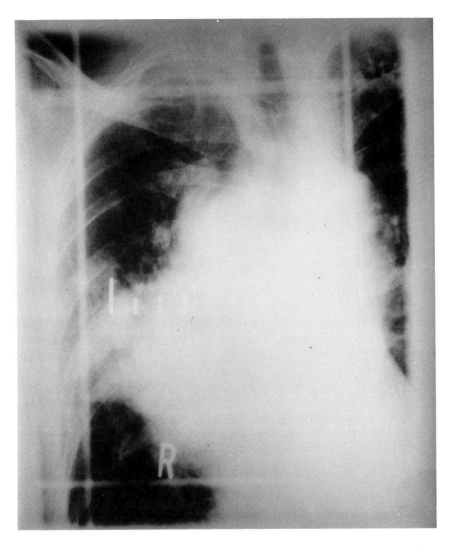

necessary to recheck the localisation, or if the marks on the patient which define the treatment area are lost.

Sealed sources

Implanted sources can be verified with the simulator. An example of this is for an Ir^{192} implant into the breast. The guide tubes, which are positioned

141

in the breast before the radioactive wires (Ir^{192}) are loaded, can be checked by using the simulator.

The breast area is screened until the beads at the edges of the guide tubes, containing dummy wires, are superimposed and a radiograph taken (see Figure 6.5). Another radiograph is then taken at 90° from the first image (see Figure 6.6). These radiographs help to demonstrate the depth of the dummy wires under the surface of the breast, and how far apart the

Figure 6.5: Radiograph showing beads superimposed. (Courtesy of Ann Hayward, Hammersmith Hospital Radiotherapy Department.)

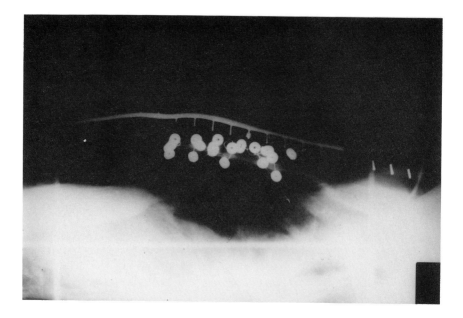

wires are positioned (single plane implant only), so the dosimetry for the area can be calculated. This means that if the dummy guide wires are badly aligned, and the area is not going to receive the prescribed amount of radiation, then the guide tubes can be moved before the radioactive wires are loaded.

For a double plane implant it is a little more difficult to line up the beads successfully, and it may be necessary to use diagnostic tomography.[11]

Figure 6.6: Radiograph showing guide wires and beads. (Courtesy of Ann Hayward, Hammersmith Hospital Radiotherapy Department.)

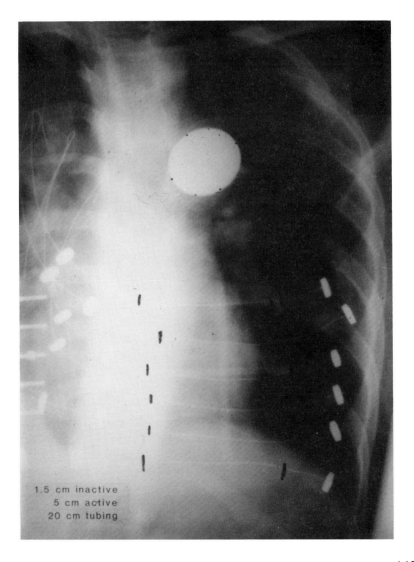

1.5 cm inactive
5 cm active
20 cm tubing

RADIOLOGICAL CONTRAST MEDIA

Radiological contrast media (referred to in the text as contrast media) are used for some localising procedures with the simulator (see below), and only contrast media relevant to use with the simulator will be discussed (for more information see Chapman and Nakielny, Further Reading). They demonstrate parts of the body — for instance, kidneys, oesophagus and bladder (see Figure 6.7), which would not normally be outlined clearly

Figure 6.7: Radiograph showing contrast medium in the bladder; AP pelvis. (Courtesy of the Middlesex Hospital Radiotherapy Department.)

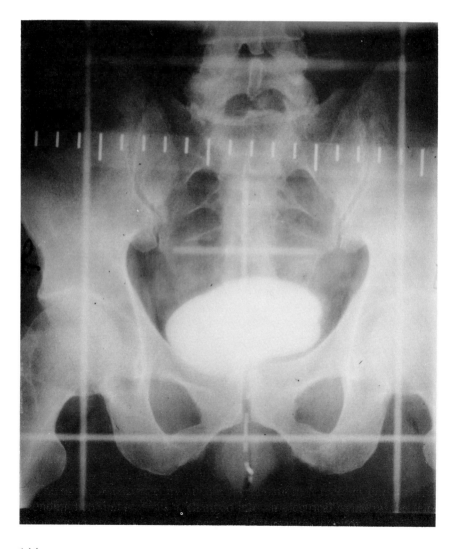

when producing conventional radiographs (without using contrast media). The contrast media can be classified as negative or positive.

Negative contrast media

These have a low atomic number and are radiolucent (do not readily absorb radiation at the energies used with the simulator). Substances such as carbon dioxide, oxygen and air are used as negative contrast media, and will show on the radiograph as a dark area.

Positive contrast media

These have a high atomic number, are radio-opaque (readily absorb radiation at the energies used with the simulator) and show on the radiograph as a light area. Positive contrast media are in the form of barium compounds or iodine compounds.

Barium compounds

Barium would be toxic (poisonous) if it is absorbed into the blood stream,[12] so it is made into an inert salt such as barium sulphate, which is insoluble, to be used as a contrast medium. It helps to outline the gastrointestinal tract and is produced in various forms, either as a powder, in a suspension or as a paste, with different concentrations (100 per cent w/v has 1 g of barium in 100 ml of contrast medium; 50 per cent w/v has 0.5 g of barium in 100 ml of contrast medium). A higher percentage w/v means that the medium will attenuate more radiation than a medium of lower percentage w/v. Barium products are reasonably cheap, approximately 30–40p per 50 ml.

A few examples of barium products are listed below:

(1) *Baritop 100 (Concept Pharmaceuticals Ltd)*. A suspension of barium sulphate in a sealed can containing 300 ml, with a concentration of 100 per cent w/v. It should be stored in a warm place and shaken thoroughly before use.
(2) *Baritop G 97 per cent (Concept Pharmaceuticals Ltd)*. A white powder of barium sulphate which needs the appropriate quantity of water to be added for the barium concentration (percentage w/v) required. This information is shown on the instructions supplied by the manufacturer. It is then thoroughly mixed to produce a homogeneous solution.
(3) *E-Z-HD (Henley's Medical Supplies)*. Barium sulphate powder which

forms a suspension with the addition of the correct amount of water to 250 per cent w/v. To make it palatable it has additives to give a fresh fruit flavour.

(4) *E-Z-Paque (Henley's Medical Supplies).* This is barium sulphate in powder form. On the packet there is a guide to the amount of water needed for the different barium concentrations. (For 100 per cent w/v the solution is made up to 177 ml.) It also has a fresh fruit flavour.

(5) *Micropaque Liquid Dispersion (Nicholas Laboratories Ltd).* Barium sulphate in solution 95 per cent w/v.

(6) *Microtrast (Nicholas Laboratories Ltd).* Barium sulphate paste, 70 per cent w/v, a rather thick substance.

Iodine compounds

The main types of iodine compounds are the water-soluble contrast media, which can be split into ionic, ionic with low osmolarity (osmolality) and non-ionic with low osmolarity. Osmolality and osmolarity can be used as interchangeable terms for practical purposes.[3]

Osmolality

This is defined as the osmotic concentration of a fluid expressed as the number of osmols per kg of water (dissolved in 1 kg of water).

Osmolarity

This is defined as the osmotic concentration of a fluid expressed as the number of osmols of solute per litre of solution (substance and water making a total volume of 1 litre).

Iodine would also be poisonous if it were absorbed directly into the blood stream and is therefore bound to a stable 'carrier molecule' of low toxicity.

Ionic contrast media

A conventional ionic contrast medium is made up of tri-iodinated derivatives of benzoic acid.[12] The chemical structure consists of molecules which contain a benzene ring (a ring of six hydrogen atoms linked with six carbon atoms, see Figure 6.8a,b), with a carboxyl placed at one end of the benzene ring to form benzoic acid (see Figure 6.8c). Iodine replaces three hydrogen atoms of the benzene ring (see Figure 6.8d) and two more hydrogen atoms are replaced by short-chain hydrocarbons R1 and R2 (see Figure 6.8e). A typical compound formed in this manner is called iothalamic acid, and if one

Figure 6.8: Chemical structure of water-soluble contrast media. (Reproduced by permission of Dr Peter Dawson, *Radiography*, 1984, **50** (592).)

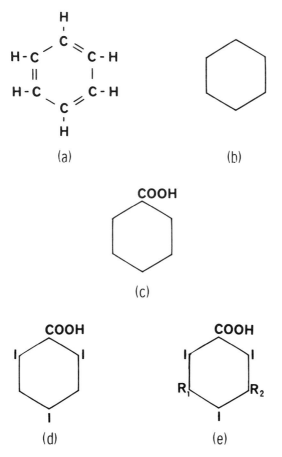

of the side chains is slightly changed diatrizoic acid is formed. The acid is turned into a salt by using sodium or meglumine for use as contrast media. A few examples of conventional ionic contrast media are listed below.

(1) *Conray 420 (May and Baker)*. This is sodium iothalamate prepared in solution of 420 mg/ml of iodine.
(2) *Conray 280 (May and Baker)*. Meglumine iothalamate which has 280 mg/ml iodine.
(3) *Hypaque 25 per cent (Winthrop Laboratories)*. Sodium diatrizoate with 150 mg of iodine per ml. Hypaque 45 per cent contains 270 mg iodine per ml.
(4) *Urografin 150 (Schering)*. Contains 146 mg of iodine per ml and is

made up of meglumine diatrizoate 26.1 per cent w/v and sodium diatrizoate 3.9 per cent w/v.

(5) *Urografin 290 (Schering).* Contains 292 mg of iodine per ml and is meglumine diatrizoate 52.1 per cent w/v and sodium diatrizoate 7.9 per cent w/v.

(The above examples are usually administered intravenously or via a catheter, for example, into the bladder. They are obtainable in different amounts; the smallest is a 20 ml ampoule and the price of 20 ml varies from 80p to £1.30 (1986/7 list prices) depending on the concentration of the contrast medium.)

(6) *Gastrografin (Schering).* The iodine content is 370 mg per ml, and is made up of 10 per cent sodium diatrizoate and 66 per cent meglumine diatrizoate in solution, with added flavouring which gives an aniseed taste. This product is administered orally and is produced in 100 ml bottles (5 × 100 ml £24.50, 1986/7 price).

Action of ionic contrast media

When an ionic contrast medium is introduced into solution it will ionise.[13,14] The sodium and meglumine salts form positive ions. These are not radiologically useful and may be clinically toxic to the patient.[15] The iodinated benzoate is left as the negative ion, which is of radiological value. Ionic contrast media has five to eight times the osmolarity of blood plasma, and this is also related to some of the side-effects caused by contrast media.[13,14]

Adverse effects related to osmolarity

Cells behave differently when exposed to solutions of different osmolarity. If extracellular fluid is hypo-osmolar the cell will take in water because of osmosis. However, if the extracellular fluid is hyperosmolar water is drawn out of the cell by osmosis.

When hyperosmolar substances are introduced into the blood plasma, as is the case with ionic contrast media, water is drawn out from the cells and they shrink and distort.[13] This happens mainly to the endothelial cells, red cells, white cells and platelets. If the endothelial cells are badly damaged there is a risk of thrombosis, and damage to the white cells leads to a histamine release and a variety of side-effects (see below). The blood volume will increase because of the extra fluid from the cells, and may cause a change in cardiac output.

High osmolarity is not the total cause of all the side-effects, but seems to play a major role. This is a good reason for trying to reduce osmolarity by using low osmolar compounds.

Non-ionic contrast media with low osmolarity

Osmolarity is proportional to the number of particles in solution. The molecules of the ionic compounds dissociate into two particles, a positive and a negative ion. If the molecules should give only one particle in the solution, this will reduce the osmolarity.[12] This is achieved by using a non-ionic contrast medium.

This is made up of a tri-iodinated benzoic acid derivative, with the carboxyl group on the benzene ring, as in the structure of a ionic contrast medium, replaced by a side chain R3 (see Figure 6.9). Non-ionic contrast media are prepared as iohexol or iopamidol. They do not ionise in solution and have low osmolarity.[12]

(1) *Omnipaque (Nycomed — Nyegaard).* This is iohexol and is produced in various concentrations of iodine content: 180 mg I/ml, 240 mg I/ml, 300 mg I/ml and 350 mg I/ml.
(2) *Niopam (Merck — Bracco Ltd, Milan).* Prepared as iopamidol in the various forms: 200 mg I/ml, 300 mg I/ml and 370 mg I/ml.

They are generally administered intravenously and produced in different quantities (20 ml, 50 ml, 100 ml). The cost of the non-ionic contrast media (20 ml) ranges from £5 to £8 (1986/7 list prices).

Ionic contrast media with low osmolarity

When two tri-iodinated benzoic acid derivatives are linked together and a carboxyl group is replaced by a side-chain R3 (see Figure 6.10) an ionic contrast medium with low osmolarity is formed. This is prepared as sodium

Figure 6.9: Chemical structure of a non-ionic compound. (Reproduced by permission of Dr Peter Dawson, *Radiography*, 1984, **50** (592).)

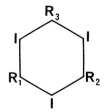

Figure 6.10: Chemical structure of an ionic compound with low osmolarity. (Reproduced by permission of Dr Peter Dawson, *Radiography*, 1984, **50** (592).)

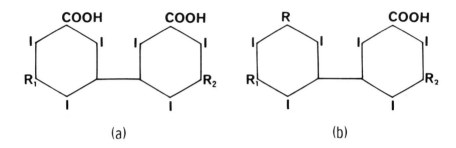

meglumine ioxaglate (Hexabrix). Each molecule will dissociate into two particles, but as there are six iodines per molecule instead of three, only half the number of molecules are required for the same iodine concentration as with the conventional ionic medium. This means that the osmolarity is effectively reduced.[12]

Hexabrix 320 (May and Baker)

This is a clear pale yellow solution containing 320 mg per ml of iodine and 39.3 per cent w/v meglumine ioxaglate and 19.65 per cent w/v sodium ioxaglate. Hexabrix can be administered intravenously and is made up in varying amounts. The cost of 20 ml is approximately £3.50 (1986/7 list price).

Ideal contrast media

Non-toxic — not poisonous.
Inert — stable chemically.
Low viscosity — low resistance to flow when introduced into the body.
Low osmolarity — reduces hyperosmolarity of body fluids.
Rapidly excreted — removed quickly from the body.
Non-carcinogenic — does not cause cancer.

The ideal contrast medium unfortunately has not yet been produced by the manufacturers, and reactions to the contrast media can vary from minimal to extremely severe (see below). The tolerance of the patient to possible side-effects depends on the volume, concentration and speed with which the contrast medium is administered. A small volume, of low concentration, introduced slowly, will give fewest side-effects but a compromise has to be made to ensure that the contrast medium is radiologically useful.

When an iodinated contrast medium is introduced intravenously the procedure carries a risk to the patient. There is an increased risk of a reaction, to the contrast medium, in patients with any of the following conditions:

Hypersensitivity to iodine
Thyrotoxicosis
Previous severe reaction
Cardiac and coronary disease
Severe respiratory disease
Hepatico-renal syndrome (hepatic and renal failure)
Pregnancy — teratogenic effect

Contrast media should not be given intravenously to patients undergoing plasma protein and radioisotope tests as cell function is inhibited by the contrast media.[16]

Reactions to iodinated contrast media when given intravenously

Minor reactions

These require no drug treatment but firm reassurance and explanation of the procedure to lessen the anxiety for the patient.[16] Some of the reactions a patient may experience are: nausea, vomiting, feeling of heat, pallor, sweating, coughing, sneezing, metallic taste.

Allergic reactions

Antihistamine drugs may be given to counteract these reactions.[16] The reactions can include: flushing of the skin; sore, watering eyes; urticarial rash.

Acute anaphylaxis

This is a severe allergic reaction which can occur within minutes of administering the contrast medium.[16] Acute anaphylaxis can cause: severe shortness of breath, sweating, rapid pulse, fall in blood pressure, circulatory collapse.

The patient may die unless immediate measures are taken.

Moderate reactions

These require some drug treatment[16] such as antihistamines with simple first aid (see *St John First Aid Manual*, Further Reading). The following are moderate reactions which patients may experience during this procedure: severe vomiting, extensive urticaria, oedema of the face and glottis, dyspnoea, rigors, pains in the chest and abdomen, fainting.

Severe reactions

Any of the following are severe reactions[16]: loss of consciousness, pulmonary oedema, myocardial infarction, cardiac arrhythmias, cardiac arrest.

These types of reactions require intensive treatment with drugs, and cardiac and respiratory resuscitation where applicable.

If administering iodinated contrast media intravenously it is therefore necessary to have certain equipment and drugs within the near proximity.[16] A list of these items is given below:

(1) *Emergency equipment*: piped oxygen or oxygen cylinder with tubing and mask; suction apparatus and catheter; laryngoscope, endotracheal tubes; Brooks airway; ventilation bag (Ambu bag); needles and syringes, intravenous giving set; scalpel blade; stethoscope and sphygmomanometer.

(2) *Emergency drugs*: piriton — antihistamine; hydrocortisone — anti-inflammatory; adrenaline — increase cardiac output; aminophylline — stimulates muscular tissue of the heart; nikethamide — respiratory stimulant; atropine — for bradycardia after myocardial infarction; lignocaine — reduces excitability of heart muscle; sodium bicarbonate — corrects metabolic acidosis; calcium chloride — restores heart tone; dextrose — fluid replacement; diazepam — for anxiety; frusemide — diuretic; saline; water for injection.

Pros and cons for using low osmolar contrast media

The reaction rate to conventional ionic contrast media is 4 per cent of the general population. In those with an already known allergy the rate is 10–12 per cent and if they have had a previous reaction, 15–6 per cent. The mortality rate due to ionic contrast media in intravenous urography (a contrast medium injected intravenously to image the kidneys) is estimated at 1 in 10,000 to 1 in 40,000.

A study over one year was undertaken to monitor a non-ionic low osmolar contrast medium, Omnipaque, when used for urography. There were 50,660 patients in the trial and it was shown that 97.9 per cent of the patients had no adverse reactions and there were no fatalities.[17] It has been indicated that more reactions have been experienced with the low osmolar ionic contrast medium (Hexabrix), when injected intravenously than the non-ionic contrast media.[12]

The conventional ionic contrast media, when administered intravenously, are reasonably safe, but are associated with a variety of side-effects which patients find distressing. The newer low osmolar contrast media have fewer side effects but are four to six times more expensive, at present.

These non-ionic low osmolar contrast media are useful for patients who have had a previous reaction or allergy, a debilitated patient, a patient with renal failure, an elderly patient or an infant.

LOCALISING PROCEDURES USING RADIOLOGICAL CONTRAST MEDIA

It is important that the contrast medium to be used is checked by two people, ensuring that it is the correct contrast medium, correct strength and volume, and that the contents are as expected. The expiry date should also be noted, and if the contrast medium is to be used in an aseptic situation check that the seal is not damaged, before it is broken for use.

Oesophagus

To visualise the oesophagus using the simulator for localisation it is helpful to use barium sulphate in suspension or Gastrografin as a contrast medium. Currently non-ionic contrast media are being used for this procedure as they are more easily absorbed into the surrounding tissue than the barium, if there is a perforation of the oesophagus. (See different types of contrast media at the beginning of this chapter.)

The contrast medium is given orally and the reactions are not usually severe, but sometimes nausea or vomiting may be experienced by the patient. Only a small amount of contrast medium is required, about 50 ml. A cup with a spout or bendable straw is useful for the patient to take the fluid.

Procedure

The patient is placed supine on the simulator couch with hands extended away from the thorax, usually behind the head, and the approximate area for treatment positioned using the optical light beam. The patient is given a few sips of contrast medium and then asked to hold a mouthful. When the patient is told to swallow, the passage of the barium can be watched during fluoroscopy on the television monitor. This will show any obstruction or displacement of the oesophagus.

The area for treatment can now be positioned more accurately than if a contrast medium was not used. The same procedure is now followed as for localisation of a radical treatment (see earlier in this chapter) and an AP and lateral radiograph can be taken as the patient swallows more contrast medium. The exposure factors are similar for an image of the chest (see

General guide to exposure factors, earlier in this chapter) but a higher kV will help to penetrate the mediastinum and to define the area around the contrast medium.

After the localisation procedure is completed the patient should be given water to drink, to remove any remaining contrast medium in the mouth, and paper tissues to remove excess around the mouth.

Bladder

The patient is catheterised using an aseptic technique,[18,19] for this localising procedure with a contrast medium.

After emptying the bladder 40 ml of water-soluble iodinated contrast medium is introduced into the bladder via the catheter, plus 5–10 ml of air. (See the different types of contrast media at the beginning of this chapter.) As the contrast medium will be expelled after the procedure via the catheter the patient does not suffer reactions from the contrast medium.

The patient is positioned supine with hands on the chest and the approximate centre aligned with the light beam centre. This is screened to find the borders of the treatment field and the usual procedure followed as for localisation for a radical treatment (see earlier in this chapter).

The AP radiograph will show only the positive contrast medium in the pelvis depicting the area of the bladder. The lateral radiograph will show both the positive and negative contrast medium in the bladder. The air (negative contrast medium) which rises to the surface of the bladder will define the anterior wall of the bladder. The information gained from these radiographs will help with the positioning of the target volume on the cross-sectional outline (see above).

When the procedure is finished the contrast medium is expelled from the bladder via the catheter and the catheter removed.

Some radiotherapy departments prefer to use a CT scanner to localise the bladder, and catheterisation of the patient is not needed (see Chapter 7).

Prostate

A similar localisation procedure is used as above. The patient needs to be catheterised but it is important to use a Foley catheter,[20] so that about 10 ml of water-soluble iodinated contrast medium is injected into the balloon of the catheter, as well as the usual amount (40 ml) into the bladder. When the catheter is inserted and the balloon inflated it is gently positioned so that the balloon sits at the neck of the bladder. This is where the prostate is situated, and the prominent circular area of the balloon will be easily identifiable on an image. After positioning and fluoroscopy an AP radiograph is taken (see earlier in the chapter).

A vital structure close to the prostate is the rectum, and it is important to be able to locate the rectum in relation to the target area for treatment. The dose to the rectum can then be worked out to ensure it is within tolerable limits. Before the lateral radiograph is taken a small amount of contrast medium can be put into the rectum. Barium sulphate in suspension, 20–30 ml, is slowly and gently injected via a separate catheter into the rectum.[20] The area of the rectum will then be seen more clearly on the lateral radiograph, as well as the prostate and bladder. The localisation continues as for a radical treatment (see earlier).

When the procedure is finished the catheter in the bladder is removed, after deflating the balloon, and the catheter from the rectum taken out.

Kidney shielding

When treating patients with radiotherapy in close proximity to the kidneys it is important that these vital structures are located. This is so that they can be shielded, by using lead blocks in a special carrier on the treatment unit. It will ensure the kidneys do not receive a radiation dose above their tolerance limit. To be able to see the kidneys clearly on a radiograph it is necessary to give intravenous water-soluble iodinated contrast media (see different types of contrast media at the beginning of this chapter).

Localising procedure

It is important that the medical officer asks about any allergies or previous reactions to contrast media before this procedure takes place, as the patient can experience from minor to severe reactions (see earlier in this chapter). It is useful to be able to use non-ionic contrast media (see earlier in this chapter) if available, as the reaction rate is minimal.

The patient is positioned, for the technique related to the treatment, on the simulator couch. It is helpful to warm the contrast medium to body temperature before it is injected, as this will make it less viscous. An aseptic procedure should be used at the needle site, which is usually into a vein in the antecubital fossa. Generally 40 ml of iodinated water-soluble contrast medium is then slowly injected to try to lessen side-effects. The medical officer should be present at all times during this procedure, as reactions are not always instantaneous, and the emergency drugs and equipment should be readily available (see earlier in this chapter).

When the contrast medium reaches the kidneys it goes to the glomeruli, and is filtered with water and electrolytes into the nephrons. At this point the concentration of contrast medium in the filtrate is very low, and the kidneys will not be clearly defined on a radiograph. The solute containing the contrast medium carries on passing through the tubules of the nephrons towards the collecting tubules. Most of the water has now been reabsorbed back into the blood, and there is a high concentration of contrast medium. This passes with the urine into the calyces, renal pelvis and down the ureters to the bladder to be excreted.[21]

It is usual to take an AP radiograph of this area immediately; although the concentration of contrast medium will be low an outline of the kidneys can be seen. This is important as the image shows the whole of the kidneys rather than just the calyces and renal pelvis, which are seen more clearly about five minutes after the contrast medium is injected.

The area for shielding is marked on the radiograph, which can either be used to make specialised alloy shielding blocks,[22] or by using fluoroscopy and lead markers the area from the radiograph can be transposed onto the patient. A template is then produced for treatment purposes with another AP radiograph, for verification, showing the lead markers.

When the procedure is completed the medical officer should make sure the patient is fit enough to be allowed to travel home, or to the ward if the patient is staying in hospital. (For more details of these localising techniques see Bentel *et al.*, Bleehen *et al.* and Dobbs and Barrett, Further Reading).

REFERENCES

1. Dobbs, J. and Barrett, A. (1985) *Practical Radiotherapy Planning, Royal Marsden Hospital Practice*, Edward Arnold, London, pp. 4-5.
2. Watkins, D.M.B. (1981) *Radiation Therapy Mold Technology*, Pergamon Press, Oxford, pp. 62-7.
3. Bleehen, N.M., Glatstein, E. and Haybittle, J.L. (1983) *Radiation Therapy Planning*, Marcel Dekker, New York, pp. 88-94.
4. Mould, R.F. (1981) *Radiotherapy Treatment Planning*, Adam and Hilger, Bristol, pp. 152-63
5. Bleehen, N.M., Glatstein, E. and Haybittle, J.L. (1983) *Radiation Therapy Planning*, Marcel Dekker, New York, pp. 181-263.
6. Watkins, D.M.B. (1981) *Radiation Therapy Mold Technology*, Pergamon Press, Oxford, pp. 7-18.
7. Dobbs, J. and Barrett, A. (1985) *Practical Radiotherapy Planning*, Edward Arnold, London, p. 3.
8. Kodak, 'Radiographic quality', *Fundamentals of Radiographic Photography*, vol. III, pp. 16-17.
9. Wilks, R. (1981) *Principles of Radiological Physics*, Churchill Livingstone, Edinburgh, pp. 39-47.
10. Watkins, D.M.B. (1981) *Radiation Therapy Mold Technology*, Pergamon Press, Oxford, pp. 19-32, 44-8.
11. Bleehen, N.M., Glatstein, E. and Haybittle, J.L. (1983) *Radiation Therapy Planning*, Marcel Dekker, New York, pp. 470-7.
12. Dawson, P. (1984) 'Contrast agents: a review of low osmolarity media', *Radiography*, **50**(592), 142-5.

13. Grainger, R.G. (1980) 'Osmolality of intravascular radiological contrast media', *British Journal of Radiology*, **53**, 739-46.
14. Dawson, P. (1983) 'The new low osmolar contrast media: a simple guide', *Clinical Radiology*, **34**, 221-6.
15. Chapman, S. and Nakielny, R. (1981) *A Guide to Radiological Procedures*, Baillière Tindall, London, p. 63.
16. Chapman, S. and Nakielny, R. (1981) *Guide to Radiological Procedures*, Baillière Tindall, London, pp. 2-3, 233, 236-7.
17. Schrott, K.M., Behrends, B., Clauss, W., *et al.* (1986) 'Iohexol in excretory urography', *Fortschritte der Medizin*, **104**, 153-6.
18. Lockhead, J.N.M. (1983) *Care of the Patient in Radiotherapy*, Blackwell Scientific Publications, Oxford, pp. 85-6.
19. Ehrlich, R.A. and Givens, E.M. (1985) *Patient Care in Radiography*, 2nd edn, C.V. Mosby Co., New York, pp. 183-8.
20. Gunn, C. and Tozer, C. (1982) *Guidelines on Patient Care in Radiography*, Churchill Livingstone, Edinburgh, pp. 156-8.
21. Winthrop, *Radiographers' Handbook*, Winthrop Laboratories, pp. 1-3.
22. Watkins, D.M.B. (1981) *Radiation Therapy Mold Technology*, Pergamon Press, Oxford, pp. 92-9.

Private communications

A. Hayward; S. Henman (Nyegaard); J. Stock; M. Viljoen; Guy's Schools of Radiography and Radiotherapy; Middlesex Hospital Imaging Department; Middlesex Hospital Radiotherapy Department.

Manufacturers' literature

Micropaque, barium sulphate for diagnostic radiology of the gastrointestinal tract, Nicholas Laboratories Ltd.
Water-soluble contrast media, Conray contrast media, May and Baker.
Low osmolar contrast media, a comparison with Hexabrix 320, May and Baker.
Diagnostic product information urographic and angiographic media, Schering.
Non-ionic contrast media Omnipaque, Nyegaard.
Niopam, the medium of the future, Merck.

FURTHER READING

Bentel, G.C. Nelson, C.E. and Noell, K.T. (1982) *Treatment Planning and Dose Calculation in Radiation Oncology*, 3rd edn, Pergamon Press, New York.
Bleehen, N.M., Glatstein, E. and Haybittle, J.L. (1983) *Radiation Therapy Planning*, Marcel Dekker, New York.
Chapman, S. and Nakielny, R. (1981) *A Guide to Radiological Procedures*, Baillière Tindall, London.
Dobbs, J. and Barrett, A. (1985) *Practical Radiotherapy Planning*, Edward Arnold, London.
St John Ambulance (1982) *St John First Aid Manual*, Dorling Kindersley Ltd, London.

7

Computed Tomography and Transverse Analogue Tomography
(as aids for radiotherapy planning)

COMPUTED TOMOGRAPHY

Computed tomography is also known as computerised axial tomography. It shows cross-sectional slices of varying widths through the patient, and is capable of demonstrating soft tissue clearly (see Figure 7.1). This information is useful in localising the tumour volume and obtaining transverse outlines (see Chapter 6) for radiotherapy planning.

CT scanner

A CT scanner is used for computed tomography. It produces a well-defined beam of X-rays, which is attenuated as it passes through the patient, and is then incident on an array of electronic detectors. These take readings of the emerging radiation from the patient and this information is processed by a computer. The reconstruction of a cross-section through the patient can then be viewed on a television monitor (see Chapter 5).

Original CT scanner

This was invented by Godfrey Hounsfield of EMI in 1967 and the first operational scanner was used in 1971.

First-generation scanner

This consisted of a gantry with a stationary anode X-ray tube and opposite this a single detector.[1] A pencil beam of X-rays was produced as the gantry made a linear traverse (translation) and the detector received the attenuated radiation. The gantry then rotated (indexed) through one degree, and another linear traverse was made, during which readings were taken by the detector (see Figure 7.2). This procedure continued until the gantry had rotated through 180°. The scan time was approximately five minutes, and five minutes for processing through the computer (see below). The scanner was used only for head scans.

Figure 7.1: CT scan — section through pelvis. (Courtesy of Dr Jane Dobbs, Royal Marsden Hospital Department of Radiotherapy and Oncology.)

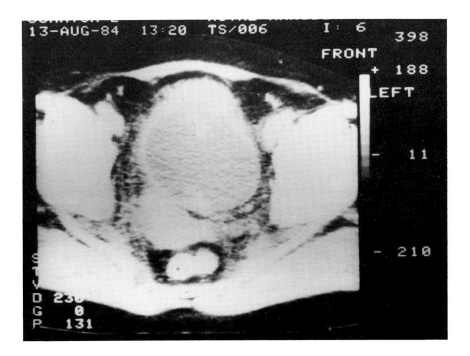

Second-generation scanner

This was called a translate-and-rotate, fan beam scanner. Instead of one detector there were up to 30 arranged in a fan opposite the X-ray tube. For each translation and rotation similar to the first-generation scanner a number of readings were taken, but because of the greater number of detectors less rotations were needed. This means that scan times were made shorter: for a scanner with eight detectors a 1-minute scan per slice and with 30 detectors, 20 seconds for a scan. As a shorter time had been achieved it was now possible to produce reasonable body scans. The problem with slow scans is that any involuntary movement of the patient produces artefacts which degrade the image.

Third-generation scanner

The third-generation scanner is the most common type of scanner in use today. It has a rotate/rotate system with an extended fan of detectors. The detectors are mounted opposite the X-ray tube so that they rotate simultaneously and there is no lateral movement of the gantry. It is necessary to rotate between 220° and 360° around the patient for a useful image to be reconstructed. The scan time for one cross-sectional slice can be cut down to two seconds.

Fourth-generation scanner

This is a rotate and stationary system and is also called a ring detector system. The X-ray tube rotates around the patient inside a circle of stationary detectors. The time for a scan of 360° is the same as for the third-generation scanners.

Radiation dose

The third- and fourth-generation scanners will give a radiation dose of 1–5 cGy to each slice of the patient.

Figure 7.2: Schematic arrangement of early CT scanners. (Reproduced by permission of Kodak Ltd.)

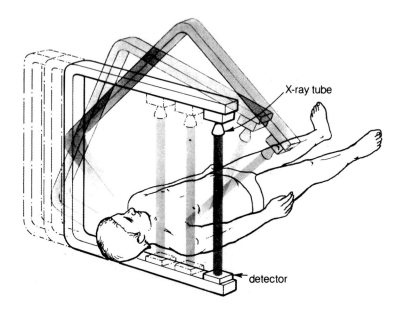

EQUIPMENT OF A MODERN CT SCANNER (see Figure 7.3)

Gantry

This is a support mechanism containing the X-ray tube and detectors. It has an aperture for the couch to move through, with a diameter up to 70 cm now available.

X-ray system

This consists of an X-ray tube, usually a rotating anode tube, with a focal spot which can be from 0.6 to 1.6 mm^2. To produce the power a generator with three-phase twelve-pulse or constant potential is required.[2,3] The exposure needed from the generator is between 120 and 140 kV and 200–1000 mAs. The X-ray beam is collimated at the tube end and the detector end, to define the beam and also to improve the image by removing scatter.

Detectors

In the modern scanners these are either scintillation crystals (cadmium tungstate) with solid-state photodiodes, or gas detectors which contain xenon at several atmospheres pressure with an electrode assembly.[2,3] An expensive CT scanner may have up to 700 detectors.

Couch

This must be strong, rigid and capable of holding large patients, as it will travel through the gantry aperture and may not be fully supported on the other side of the gantry. The couch is radiolucent so that it does not produce artefacts which would degrade the image.

Computer system

The computer system will control the file management, for example, putting in the patient data, and the scanning parameters such as kV, mA/mAs, time and slice thickness. It also controls scanning of the patient and reconstructing the image.

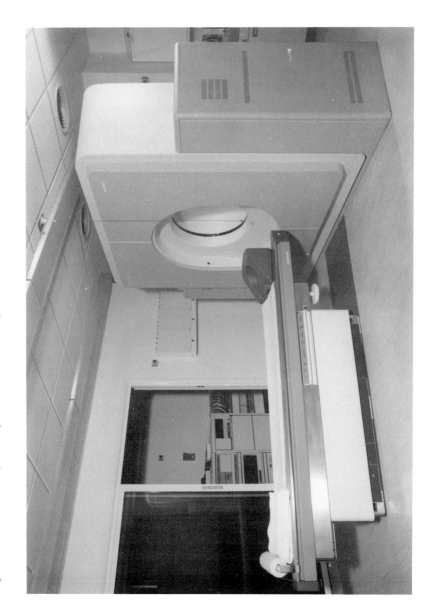

Figure 7.3: CT scanner. (Courtesy of Siemens Medical.)

RECONSTRUCTION OF THE IMAGE

Mathematical methods are used for reconstruction of the image with the CT scanner. The original EMI scanner used the iterative method, where the computer compares assumptions with measured values, finds the difference and corrects. The more modern scanners use analytical methods such as filtered back projection.[2-4]

The readings taken from the detectors are transferred to a computer which reconstructs the image. The signal is initially an analogue signal (continuous) which is converted to a digital signal (numerical, finite) for use with the computer. These readings are average linear attenuation coefficients of the different tissues through which the X-ray beam has passed. (The total linear attenuation coefficient is the fraction of X-rays removed from the beam per unit thickness of a medium.[5])

The stored digital image data are then processed into an analogue signal, by a digital-to-analogue converter, so that the image can be viewed on a television monitor. The time taken to reconstruct the image varies from five to 30 seconds depending on the type of scanner and the scan performed.

CT image

The image is made up of a matrix, a grid pattern as seen in Figure 7.4a. Each square on the matrix represents a   block of tissue, the voxel.

Figure 7.4a: Diagram of an 80 × 80 matrix. (Courtesy of Agfa Gevaert.)

Figure 7.4b: Diagram of a voxel 3 × 13mm. (Courtesy of Agfa Gevaert.)

Figure 7.4c: Diagram of a pixel 3 × 3 mm. (Courtesy of Agfa Gevaert.)

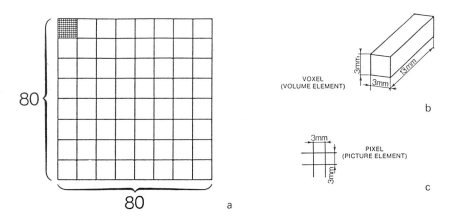

Voxel

This is the basic unit of CT reconstruction and is the volume element which is three-dimensional. It has length, width and depth of $3 \times 3 \times 13$ mm (see Figure 7.4b). The depth is determined by the thickness of the cross-sectional slice. The voxel is displayed on the television monitor in a two-dimensional image as a pixel.

Pixel

This shows width and length and is called the picture element (see Figure 7.4c). The value of each pixel is the average attenuation for the complete block of tissue the voxel.

When the first-generation scanners were used the image was reconstructed and displayed on an 80×80 matrix as shown in Figure 7.4a. The more modern scanners commonly use 256×256 or 512×512 matrices.

Hounsfield unit (HU)

This is a number, sometimes called a CT number, which is the basic unit of the CT scale. A Hounsfield unit is allotted to each individual pixel. It is derived from the relationship of the linear attenuation coefficient of the irradiated substance to the linear attenuation coefficient of water,[2] so that water is a set standard of zero on the scale and air is -1000. The scale then extends with the newer scanners to $+4000$ for the rest of the tissues in the body, bone having the higher CT numbers and soft tissue the lower CT numbers.

To show contrast on the CT image only part of the range is selected and is called the window width. If all the CT numbers are shown then the contrast of the image is not perceived by the eye as the density differences are so small. This means a narrow window width gives higher contrast on the image than a wide window width; however, the range of CT numbers used should be large enough to produce the information required.

The window width may consist of 400 HU, for example, from $+240$ to -160, and any numbers above the upper limit will show as white, and below the lower limit as black. The central HU of this window width, $+40$, is called the window level. This range ($+240$ to -160) of HU is commonly used when scanning the abdomen.

As the television monitor, on which the image is viewed, can only differentiate between 10 to 15 shades of grey the 400 HU, as in the above example, are divided into groups of 40 HU. Each group is represented by one level of grey and the image is therefore shown by a grey scale from light through to dark (see Figure 7.1).

STORING AND DISPLAYING THE CT IMAGE

There are various methods for storing and displaying the reconstructed image.

Storing the digital image data

Magnetic disk (hard)

A thin rigid platter with magnetisable material on one or both sides. The disk is fragile and must be protected from dust and extremes of temperature. The data are recorded onto and read from the disk by special read/write heads which allow the magnetic data to be turned into a signal which is used by the computer.

The sets of CT scans are stored as files on the disk and can be randomly accessed. This means each file is independent of the rest and can be found almost instantaneously by the computer for viewing purposes. The disk will record from 100 to 1000 images depending on its storage capacity and the size of the matrix of the CT image. It can cost from £100 to £30,000 and is re-usable.

Floppy disk or diskette

This is a thin flexible sheet of plastic which is coated with magnetisable material on one or both sides. It is smaller than the hard disk and easily portable but must be protected in a paper or cardboard cover. The storage capacity is low; only 4–8 CT images, depending on matrix size, can be recorded on one disk. It is similar to the hard disk in that the images are recorded in separate files and can be accessed randomly. The floppy disk costs about £2 and is re-usable.

Magnetic tape

This is a plastic tape 2.5 cm wide coated with magnetisable material on one side. It must be protected in a rigid container from dust and adverse temperatures. The whole tape may be 800 m long and it is not possible to have random access to sets of CT images (a file) — only serial access. If the information required is at the end of the tape it will take longer to obtain the data than if the information is at the beginning of the tape. It can store 50–200 images depending on matrix size, but the information cannot be viewed directly from the tape; it has to be copied onto a magnetic disk and then displayed. The tape can cost about £8 and is re-usable.

Displaying the CT image

The usual method, as already mentioned, is to convert the digital image data to an analogue signal which can be used by a television monitor to display the image (see Chapter 5). It is also useful to produce a hard copy which can be kept permanently. The most common method for this process is by photographing the CT image from a television monitor onto X-ray film or photographic paper. The film or paper is then processed in the conventional way, either by manual or daylight unloading, and passed through an automatic processor (see Chapter 4). The units used for this system are called video imagers and examples are the multiformat imagers and Vidicam camera.

Multiformat imagers

These contain a small dedicated television monitor; a camera consisting of a mirror, lens and shutter system and a special cassette to hold the single-sided X-ray film (see Chapters 1 and 2). The spectral sensitivity of the film must match the light emission from the fluorescent screen of the television monitor (cathode ray tube).

When the cassette is placed in the unit the slide is removed so that the film will be exposed. During the exposure the camera moves and the television monitor and film remain stationary, so that different formats (1, 4, 9 or 12 images) can be positioned on the same film. The size of the image is altered by varying the distance of the lens system from the film. The minimum cost for these kind of units is £13,000.

Vidicam

There is a fixed format with this unit and only one image size is available. The Vidicam has a small dedicated television monitor and camera which remain stationary, and it is the X-ray film or photographic paper which moves. The film or paper is fed from a storage box at the lower end of the unit to the upper portion, and en route it is exposed by the camera which has received an image from the monitor. It travels into a receiving cassette so that it can be developed through an automatic processor. The Vidicam can cost £5000–£6000.

Laser imager 3M

The signal used by the laser imager can be either a digital or analogue signal. The infrared laser beam is optically focused to spot size, and is guided over a special laser film by several mirrors. The film is single-sided with a polyester base and has an emulsion containing silver halide crystals. The spectral sensitivity of the film matches that of the laser beam. The film is developed conventionally, and as the laser imager can be attached to a processor daylight unloading is possible. A selection can be made as to the number of images required on one film. The unit is also capable of storing images and producing copies. The approximate cost of this equipment is £44,000 (1986/7 price).

Viewing the CT scan

If X-ray film is used to record the CT image then viewing boxes are required (see Chapter 4), otherwise only normal room lighting is needed. When looking at the CT image there is a certain convention to follow; for instance, a head scan is usually viewed as if from above the head looking down the patient. When looking at the image the patient's left side will be on the viewer's left. A body scan is viewed as looking up at the patient from below — the patient's left side is on the viewer's right.

CT SCANNER USED FOR RADIOTHERAPY PLANNING

It is extremely helpful to be able to use a CT scanner to localise tumour volumes, especially those which are difficult to image conventionally with the simulator (e.g. pancreas). However, it is also important that certain modifications are made to the CT scanner for it to be of any value for radiotherapy planning.

(1) The couch must be flat-topped as for the treatment units.
(2) A large gantry aperture is needed to allow the correct treatment position for the necessary technique, for instance, when treating with the arms raised and hands on the head.
(3) Lasers are required to align the patient accurately (see Chapter 5).

Radiotherapy CT scan

The patient must be positioned on the scanner couch as for the relevant treatment technique and the lasers are used to straighten the patient.

It is necessary, if the abdomen is being localised, to prepare the patient by giving an oral contrast medium (from 200 to 400 ml of 2 per cent gastrografin or EZ CAT barium sulphate 1.7 per cent w/v), so that the bowel is opacified and not mistaken for tumour. If the contrast medium is too dense a streaking effect is viewed on the image. However, if the technique requires that the bladder must be empty for treatment then a separate procedure is needed so that the bladder is empty when scanned.

A 'scout view'

Sometimes called a topogram or scanogram, a 'scout view' is then produced of the area to be localised. This is similar to a conventional radiograph and can be an anteroposterior view (see Figure 7.5), posteroanterior view or a lateral view (see Figure 7.6) of the patient. The chosen position for the cross-sectional slices will be superimposed onto the topogram so

167

Figure 7.5: Topogram — anteroposterior view. (Courtesy of Sue Hay, Middlesex Hospital Imaging Department.)

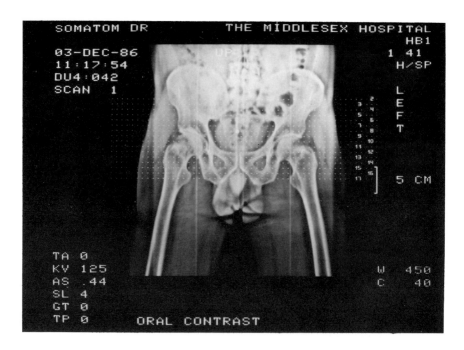

that each slice can be related to the area in the patient. The cross-sectional slices required, for example, for localising the bladder would be at 1 cm intervals from the fifth lumbar vertebra (L5) to the bottom of the obturator foramen of the pelvis and with a slice width of 8–10 mm.

Markers

These are placed on important reference points on the patient and will

Figure 7.6: Topogram — lateral view. (Courtesy of Sue Hay, Middlesex Hospital Imaging Department.)

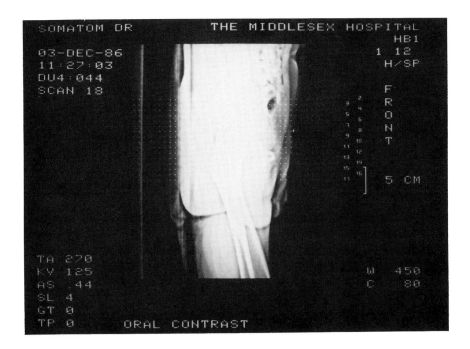

show on the topogram and cross-sectional images. The lasers are used to find these reference marks on the patient, such as the mid-line and laterally at a set distance vertically above the couch top. It is important to put an indelible mark or tattoo on the surface of the patient (see Figure 7.7) or plastic immobilisation shell which relates to where the markers are placed.

The markers are not the usual lead markers as for imaging with the simulator (see Chapter 6) but angiography catheters which are Teflon-

169

Figure 7.7: Patient positioned for therapy scan of pelvis. (Courtesy of Dr Jane Dobbs, Royal Marsden Hospital Department of Radiotherapy and Oncology.)

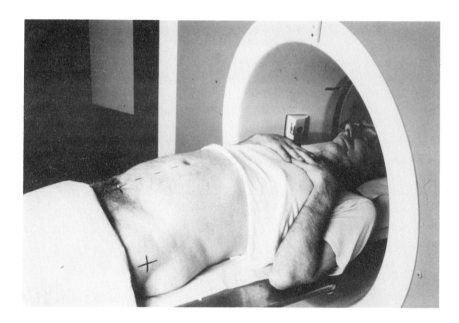

coated, or small pieces of nylon tubing packed with barium products and silicon cream. If lead were used it would produce artefacts such as streaking.

The CT images produced will help show the extent of the tumour so that the radiotherapist can decide on the target volume required for treatment. The image data are either copied onto a floppy disk, and the disk taken to the planning computer, or the data are sent directly to the computer if this option is available. (For more details on localisation techniques with the CT scanner see Reference 6.)

Scan plan

The planning computer will show the various images from the CT scanner on the console monitor (see Figure 7.8). The closest slice to the centre of the tumour volume is used to draw the target volume directly on the console monitor of the computer with a light pen (photoelectric device used to activate changes on the monitor). Any vital structures showing on the image can also be put into the computer in the same manner. Some departments prefer to use a life-size hard copy made of the central slice from the CT scanner and to draw the target volume onto this. This infor-

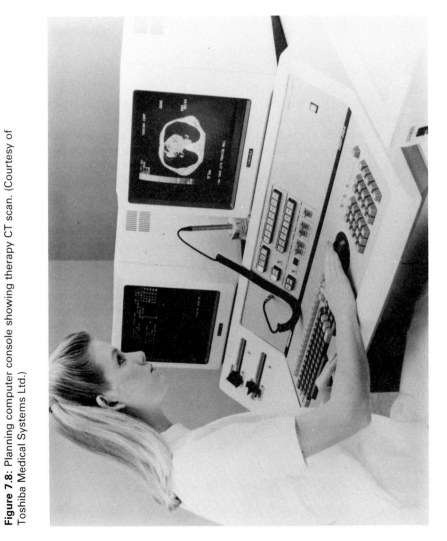

Figure 7.8: Planning computer console showing therapy CT scan. (Courtesy of Toshiba Medical Systems Ltd.)

mation is then put into the computer using a digitiser tablet[7] (see Figure 7.9).

The console monitor of the planning computer will display the dose distribution around the volume (see Figure 7.10) and pinpoint the dose to any vital structures. A hard copy can be made when the plan is satisfactory for a permanent record. (See Manufacturers' Literature for details of computer planning systems.)

Summary of advantages

The CT scans show very clearly the extent of the tumour volume as cross-sectional slices can be taken at different levels. This gives a closer approach to producing a three-dimensional image for planning rather than the two dimensions shown with conventional radiographs when using the simulator (see Chapter 6).

Soft tissue is very clearly seen, and structures such as the pancreas, kidneys and soft tissue masses in the bronchus, are easily identified. An irregular outline of the bladder, which may mean a tumour growth, and vital structures such as the spinal cord are identifiable, and this can be useful for treatment purposes. The CT scan gives excellent information on patient outline which is essential to produce a treatment plan.[8,9]

These are advantages for most radiotherapy departments but a specialised technique is performed at the Royal Free Hospital radiotherapy centre where the CT scanner has become a great asset. The procedure is three-dimensional conformational therapy, which may well be a technique used by more radiotherapy departments, as technological advances are gained for the treatment units.

Three-dimensional conformational therapy

This involves the treatment of long irregular-shaped lesions or those close to vital structures which with conventional radiotherapy would suffer unacceptable damage. The technique requires movements of the treatment unit and the patient on the treatment couch which are under computer control.[10] By using the CT scanner the planning of conformational therapy has been reduced from 2–3 hours to 30–45 minutes. This means the patient is more relaxed and the final result is an accurate plan.[11]

Summary of disadvantages

The CT scanner is expensive; it costs from £250,000 to £500,000 for the unit with running costs, including staff and maintenance, at about £100,000 per year.

Figure 7.9: Information put into planning computer using a digitiser tablet. (Courtesy of Toshiba Medical Systems Ltd.)

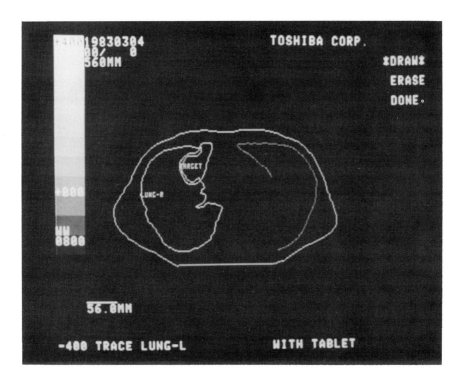

The problem of patient position with some breast techniques when using an arm pole, which protrudes at right angles to the couch, makes imaging of this area difficult. There is no attachment on the CT scanner for this accessory equipment, or room to allow it to move through the aperture of the gantry. Head and neck treatments usually involve an immobilisation shell which has a system attaching it to the couch, which again is not always possible with the CT scanner.

Localising or verifying large irregular fields is another problem for the CT scanner, and is more easily achieved with the simulator. Verification of the treatment plan is difficult as the CT scanner is unable to simulate the exact angles of the treatment plan as does the simulator (see Chapter 6).

There are perhaps only one or two radiotherapy departments which have sole use of a CT scanner, and usually time is limited for radiotherapy

Figure 7.10: Dose distribution shown around target volume using CT scan and planning computer.

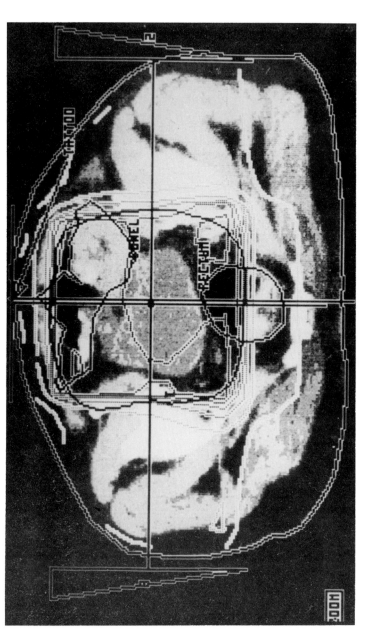

Reproduced by permission of Dobbs and Barrett (1985) *Practical Radiotherapy Planning*, Edward Arnold (Publishers) Ltd, London, p. 189.

localisation. To try to allow more time for radiotherapy some departments incorporate diagnostic scanning with radiotherapy scanning.[8,9]

TRANSVERSE ANALOGUE TOMOGRAPHY

The CT scanner is a very useful tool for radiotherapy planning. However, a system was set up to use the simulator with an image intensifier, which could produce a cross-sectional image.

Simtomix system, Oldelft

This system enables transverse analogue tomography to be performed using the Oldelft Simulix-y simulator (density differences of the cross-sectional slice are produced in analogue form[12] and not digital as with computed tomography). The unit is very similar to a conventional simulator except that it is possible to change from fluoroscopy (see Chapter 6) to transverse axial tomography, which will produce an image of a cross-sectional slice of the patient.

The Oldelft simulator has good mechanical stability and strength which will allow the equipment to keep within rigid tolerances. It has an indirect image intensifier, called the Delcalix,[12] which means the fluorescent screen is not in direct contact with the image intensifier; instead it is optically coupled by lenses or mirrors. There is a large flat input screen which produces an image with less distortion than when a direct image intensifier is used (see Chapter 5). The Delcalix system also has a scan converter which integrates and stores the signal to improve the image.[12]

To obtain the tomographic scan a powerful X-ray generator is required which is capable of producing 130 kV at 5 mA for 72 s. The focal spot of 0.3 mm^2 on the X-ray tube must also be able to withstand this exposure.[12]

The patient is positioned for the treatment technique, on the simulator couch, and the central area of the tumour volume is decided by using fluoroscopy and information from diagnostic investigations such as CT scans and plain radiographs. It is then possible to take a cross-sectional scan without moving the patient.

A well-defined beam of X-rays is produced by closing down the collimators, which happens automatically when the tomographic mode is selected. The gantry is rotated 360° around the patient and at the same time the X-rays being produced are detected by the intensifier. (More details of the tomographic scanning mode can be found in Reference 12.) To make sure there are no collisions the orientation of couch and equipment is monitored by the computer system, and any movement would be stopped if a collision were imminent.

At Chelmsford Radiotherapy and Oncology Centre, one of the departments where this unit is installed, a complete rotation of 360° takes 60 s. A circumference of 40 cm can be scanned in one rotation, but for larger areas it may be necessary to scan each half of the patient separately. The couch has inset nylon markers running longitudinally and parallel, 20 cm apart, which will not cause artefacts when seen on the image, and this allows measurements to be taken from the scan related to these marks. The dose of radiation received by the patient for one complete rotation, for instance, of the abdomen, is 0.2 cGy.

The analogue signal obtained will be immediately displayed on the television monitor, and show an image (see Figure 7.11) of the cross-sectional slice (4 mm in thickness). This electronic analogue signal can be used to produce a 'hard copy' with a Vidicam (see earlier in text) or a Video Graphic Recorder (as at Norfolk and Norwich Hospital) or stored on video cassette (see Chapter 5).

Video Graphic Recorder

The signal is applied to a fibre optic cathode ray tube face-plate. Photosensitive recording paper is passed in front of the face-plate so the image is recorded onto the paper, which is then thermally developed. This is achieved by applying an electric current directly to the carbon-backed dry silver paper. It is then cut to the appropriate size by the unit. This equipment costs about £8500 (Honeywell Video Graphic Recorder).

The analogue signal can also be put through a microprocessor unit which will digitise the information so that it can be stored on floppy disk. These image data are then used with a radiotherapy planning computer to produce a treatment plan.[12,13]

Advantages

The Simtomix is always available for radiotherapy as it is on site. The patient is not moved from treatment position as when having to go from the simulator to the CT scanner. It is easy to reproduce the treatment position for all techniques, even with an arm pole as for breast treatments. The image will give an accurate outline for the treatment plan, and bone and soft tissue structures can be identified. The cost of adding the Simtomix system to the Oldelft is about £70,000 (1986/7 price).

Disadvantages

The definition of the images is not as good as for CT scans. This unit is only installed with the Oldelft simulator.

There have been further developments to obtain better images by a company called Cynosure Limited. Their system, Cynosure 2000, produces a transaxial computed tomographic scan (digital reconstruction of the image). A conventional simulator is required, which must have an image intensifier with an input screen of 30 cm.

176

Cynosure 2000

This consists of a multi-processor computer system, operator's console, television monitor and a gantry interface, which is positioned near the gantry to record gantry movement of the simulator. (For more details see Manufacturers' Literature.)

Figure 7.11: Scan of a patient with a carcinoma of the left antrum. (Courtesy of Howard Crooks, General Hospital Cheltenham Radiotherapy and Oncology Centre.)

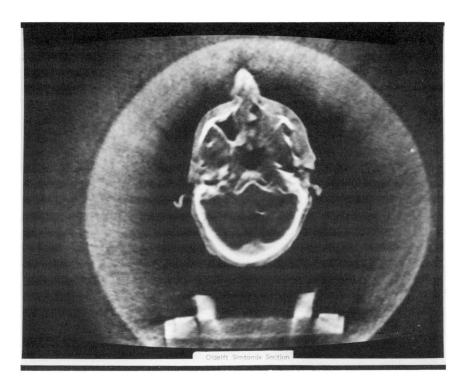

The scan is obtained by a 360° rotation with an exposure of 120 kV and 5–10 mA for 60 s and the patient receives a dose of about 0.1 cGy from a scan. A slice thickness of 2–16 mm can be chosen (for more details see Manufacturers' Literature). The digital image data received are converted to an analogue signal which can be displayed on a television monitor. The image data, in digital form, can also be transferred directly to a radiotherapy planning computer, or can be stored on floppy disk to be used with the computer.

REFERENCES

1. Kodak, 'Imaging via the cathode ray tube', *Fundamentals of Radiographic Photography*, vol. IV, section 3.
2. Curry III, T.S., Dowdey, J.E. and Murray Jr, R.C. (1984) *Christensen's Introduction to the Physics of Diagnostic Radiology*, 3rd edn, Lea and Febiger, Philadelphia, pp. 320-50.
3. Chesney, D.N. and Chesney, M.O. (1984) *X-Ray Equipment for Student Radiographers*, 3rd edn, Blackwell Scientific Publications, Oxford, pp. 458-91.
4. Gifford, D. (1984) *A Handbook of Physics for Radiologists and Radiographers*, John Wiley and Sons, Chichester, pp. 439-58.
5. Wilks, R. (1981) *Principles of Radiological Physics*, Churchill Livingstone, Edinburgh, pp. 395-412.
6. Dobbs, J. and Barrett, A. (1985) *Practical Radiotherapy Planning: Royal Marsden Hospital Practice*, Edward Arnold, London.
7. Easson, E.C. and Pointon, R.C.S. (1985) *The Radiotherapy of Malignant Disease*, Springer Verlag, Berlin, pp. 18-19.
8. Husband, J.E. and Hobday, P.A. (1981) *Computerised Axial Tomography in Oncology*, Churchill Livingstone, Edinburgh, pp. 90-100.
9. Adam, E.J., Berry, R.J., Clitherow, S. and Bedford, A. (1984) 'Evaluation of the role of computed tomography in radiotherapy treatment planning', *Clinical Radiology*, **35**, 147-50.
10. Bleehen, N.M., Glatstein, E. and Haybittle, J.L. (1983) *Radiation Therapy Planning*, Marcel Dekker, New York, pp. 139-58.
11. Tate, T. (1986) 'Conformation therapy for para-aortic metastases', *Radiography*, September, pp. 33-4.
12. Chadirchi, L.H. (1985) 'Radiotherapy planning aids on the CT body scanner at the Royal Free Hospital', *Radiography*, **51**(600), 327-9.
13. Crooks, S.H. and Hanna, F.A. (1980) 'Transverse analogue tomography in radiotherapy', *Radiography*, March, pp. 65-75.

Private communications

H. Crooks; S. Hay; M. Viljoen; Norfolk and Norwich, Radiotherapy Department.

Manufacturers' literature

Agfa Gevaert, Video Imagers.
Cynosure 2000 CT package for Transaxial Computed Tomography on Radio-
therapy Simulator Gantries, Cynosure Imaging Systems Ltd.
General Electric CT8600.
General Electric Target Radiotherapy Planning Computer.
Meditech M250 Technical Guide, Meditech Engineering Ltd.
Oldelft Simulix-y with Simtomix, Dartin Medical.
Toshiba Whole Body Scanner TCT 60AX.
Toshiba Radiotherapy Planning System TRP-02A.
Siemens Mevaplan Therapy Planning System.

FURTHER READING

Husband, J.E. and Hobday, P.A. (1981) *Computerised Axial Tomography in Oncology*, Churchill Livingstone, Edinburgh.
Redpath, A.T. and Wright, D.H. (1985) 'The use of an image processing system in radiotherapy simulation', *British Journal of Radiology*, **58**, 1081-9.

8

Ultrasound — as an aid for radiotherapy planning

Ultrasound provides detailed images of soft tissue. These images can be utilised for verification of the tumour volume, vital structures, depths in tissues and cross-sectional outlines (see Chapter 6). All this information can be of value for radiotherapy planning.

PRINCIPLES OF ULTRASOUND

Sound

This is the vibration of atoms or molecules of a substance in response to a change in pressure around the atoms or molecules. The movement to and from the particles is the quantity of vibration and is quoted as frequency (Hertz).

$$1 \text{ Hertz} = 1 \text{ oscillation per second}$$

Ultrasound is high-frequency sound waves, and for imaging purposes is usually operated in the region of 1–10 MHz.[1] Frequency determines the penetration of the wave; a high frequency means a short wavelength which gives the image better detail, but only superficial structures can be scanned. Lower frequency gives a longer wavelength which will produce images at a greater depth. The universal scanning frequency is 3.5 MHz, but it may be necessary to scan larger patients at 0.5 MHz and slim patients at 5 MHz.

To obtain a good signal (returning echo) to produce an image it is important that the tissues being scanned are of similar acoustic impedance, otherwise an acoustic boundary is formed. At an acoustic boundary some of the incident intensity of the ultrasound is reflected back and some of the intensity carries on, and so ultimately degrades the image.

Acoustic impedance

The opposition of a structure to the sound waves is its acoustic impedance. It depends on the characteristics of the tissue as to the size of the returning echo.[2]

$$\text{Acoustic impedance} = \text{density} \times \text{velocity}$$

The most valuable images using ultrasound are of soft tissue, as they have similar acoustic impedance. The velocity of ultrasound[2] in soft tissue is 1540 m/s, and so to ensure there is optimum visualisation of soft tissue a fixed velocity of 1540 m/s is used for scanning.

$$\text{Velocity} = \text{wavelength} \times \text{frequency}$$

Transducer

To produce the ultrasound and to receive the returning signal, so that the ultrasound scanner can reconstruct an image, it is necessary to use a transducer (see Figure 8.1). This emits pulses of ultrasound and also detects the reflected sound waves. The transducer is able to do this because of the piezoelectric effect of the crystal in the transducer. Basically, electrical energy is converted into sound waves (generation of ultrasound) and sound waves are converted back into electrical energy (detection of ultrasound). (For more details of the piezoelectric effect see Reference 2.)

The crystal is usually a man-made ceramic of PZT, lead-zirconium-titanate. The thickness of the crystal determines the frequency which can be obtained[2] for scanning purposes (at 3.5 MHz, crystal thickness 0.54 mm). A high voltage is needed to operate the transducer (for instance, 400 V), and induce the piezoelectric properties of the crystal, so it is important to have the transducer attached to a thick cable for insulation as it can be hand-held by the operator.

Figure 8.1: The construction of a transducer probe. (Reproduced by permission of Macmillan, London and Basingstoke (Matthew Hussey) (*Basic Physics and Technology of Medical Diagnostic Ultrasound*) p. 34. Copyright 1987 by Elsevier Science Publishing Co., Inc.)

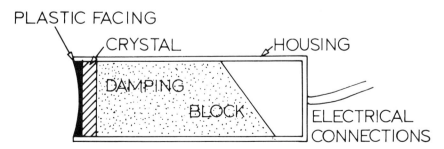

The transducer is generally a circular or rectangular shape and the front face has a plastic lens cover. This protects the crystal, provides acoustic coupling between the crystal and the skin during scanning and focuses the ultrasound beam.[2] There is a backing substance behind the crystal, generally of epoxy resin, to help dampen the pulsed ringing of the crystal[2] or else the signal becomes degraded.

The electrical signal received from the transducer is in an analogue form. This is converted to a digital signal by the computer system of the scanning unit, which will then process the information so that an image can be produced.

METHODS OF DISPLAYING THE IMAGE

The ultrasound image is generally viewed by using a television monitor (see Chapters 5 and 7). The images can be stored and viewed by using a video cassette recorder (see Chapter 5) and a hard copy made from a video imager (see Chapter 7). Recent developments enable hard copies to be produced from a video printer and thermal paper.[3] Some radiotherapy departments use a Polaroid system to obtain a hard copy.[4] The following text will briefly explain this method.

Polaroid system

A camera (Shackman, see Manufacturers' Literature) is fitted, usually to the front of the ultrasound unit. This photographs the image from a small monitor which is separate from the large monitor used for viewing.

Film unit

A pack of film units are loaded into a special attachment, on the camera, so that a hard copy can be produced. Each film unit has a negative sheet, with a silver halide emulsion, a sealed pod which contains processing chemicals and a positive sheet which has metal sulphides within a layer of cellulose. There is a black paper leader attached to the negative sheet which is also attached to a white tab which sticks out of the camera. The positive sheet is also attached to the black leader by translucent paper (see Figure 8.2a).

When packed in the film unit, the negative sheet faces the small monitor and the image is exposed onto the negative sheet. It is important to ensure the Polaroid film matches the spectral sensitivity of the phosphors used with the monitor.

Image formation

During the exposure the latent image is formed in the emulsion (see Chapter 4) of the negative sheet. The white tab is then pulled and the black leader goes through the rollers so the positive and negative sheets are

Figure 8.2a: Film pack loaded in camera back. (Courtesy of Polaroid.)

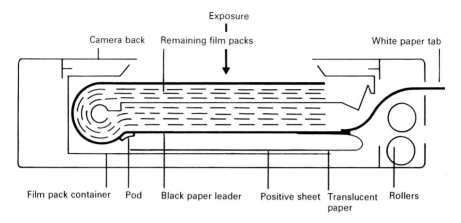

Figure 8.2b: White paper tab pulled, negative and positive sheets brought together. (Courtesy of Polaroid.)

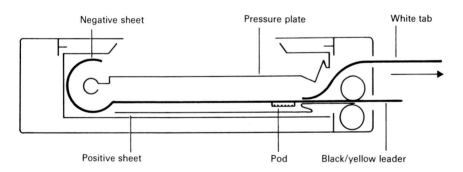

Figure 8.2c: Black leader pulled, pod ruptures to allow processing chemicals to spread between positive and negative sheets as they go between the rollers. (Courtesy of Polaroid.)

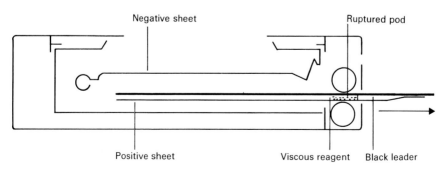

183

brought together (see Figure 8.2b). The black leader is now showing outside the camera and is steadily pulled out. The pod breaks as it passes through the rollers and the processing chemicals spread between the negative and positive sheets (see Figure 8.2c). After about 30 seconds the negative and positive sheets are pulled apart and the positive sheet shows the final image.

Development of the image

The light areas on the monitor expose the silver halide of the negative sheet which is developed by the processing chemicals. At the same time the unexposed silver halide is dissolved and transferred to the positive sheet as a soluble silver complex. This is then reduced to a silver deposit to produce the final image. No washing is required to remove the chemicals as processing agents stick to the negative sheet when it is stripped away from the positive sheet. The negative sheet can then be discarded. (For more details see Manufacturers' Literature.)

TYPES OF SCANNERS USED FOR RADIOTHERAPY PLANNING

B scanner

This has a stable T-shaped base with a vertical column and a frame which holds the small transducer. There is an electronic system for generating (with the aid of the transducer) and processing the ultrasound[5] and a display monitor for viewing the images. This kind of unit costs about £58,000 (1986/7 price).

The transducer is moved across the body to obtain the image (see Figure 8.3) and it is necessary to use the specialised oil (coupling medium oil) over the area being scanned to make good contact with the skin. This will help exclude air and prevent an acoustic boundary, so that the ultrasound is transmitted to the underlying tissue. The scan produced is called a B scan.

B scan

A visual display of a stationary image is seen as a cross-sectional slice of the area being scanned. The B scans can be used to produce the transverse outline of a patient for treatment planning (see Chapter 6) and to verify that the marks on the patient encompass the proposed area for treatment. The most useful images are from the breast, abdomen and pelvis area. (For more details of scanning the breast see Reference 6.)

However, because the B scanners are not portable and cannot be taken into the simulator (see Chapter 6) the reproducibility of patient position for treatment may be a problem. Another slight disadvantage is that as

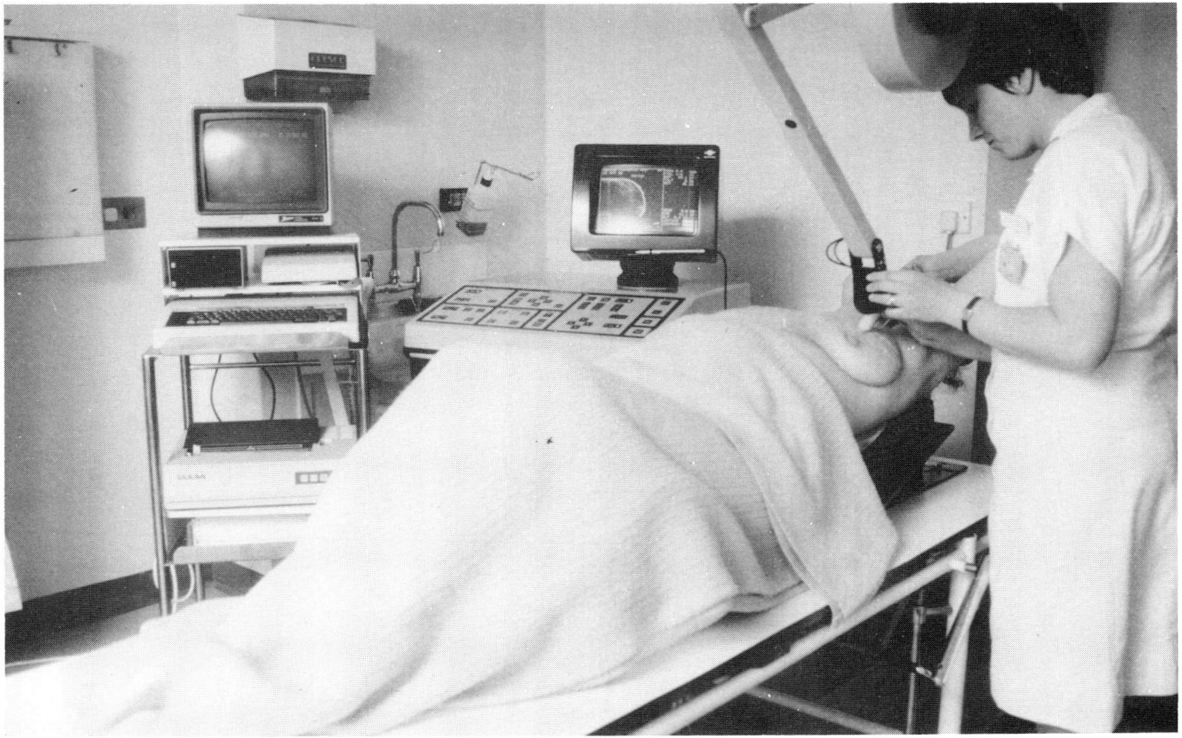

Figure 8.3: Patient in treatment position — using a B scanner to take the outline. (Reproduced by courtesy of *Radiography*, the journal of the College of Radiographers and also D. Coules and V. Lock, Bristol Radiotherapy and Oncology Centre.)

Figure 8.4: Real time scanner — Ultramark 4. (Courtesy of Scientific Medical Systems Ltd.)

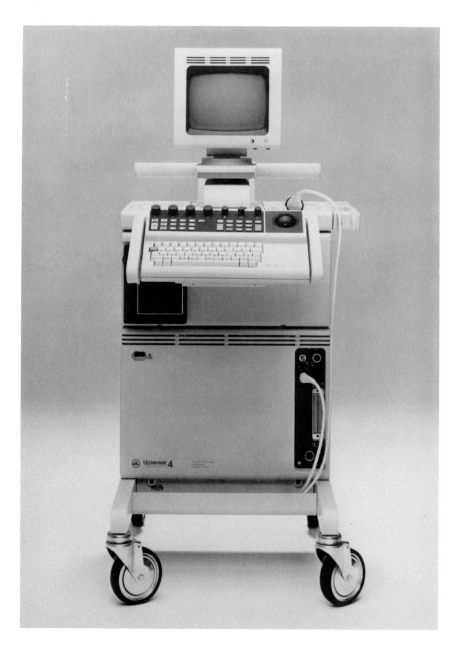

Figure 8.5: Scan of chest wall using real time scanner. The electronic marks (white crosses) in the centre of the picture show the upper and lower levels to be measured for chest wall depth. (Courtesy of Linda Harvey, Middlesex Hospital Radiotherapy Department.)

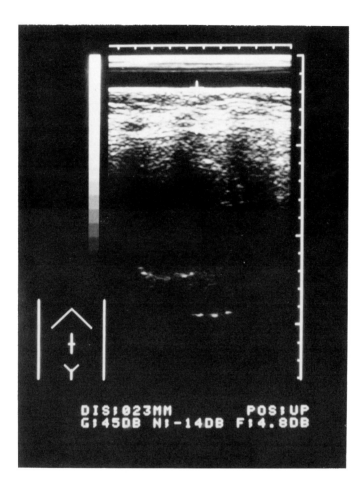

pressure is necessary to obtain good skin contact for a reasonable image, it may be possible to distort the outline.

Real time scanners

These units produce an image similar to that from the B scanner, but show movements within a scanning field. They consist of a transducer attached to a flexible cable, electronic system and display monitor (see Figure 8.4). (For more details see Reference 5.) Their cost is relatively cheap, from £5000 to the most sophisticated scanner at about £100,000. The real time scanners are easily manoeuvred. They can be used wherever there is a 240 V plug socket, and it is possible to take these units into the simulator room so that patient position can be accurately reproduced.

A useful scan is determining chest wall thickness for breast treatments, so that as much underlying lung as possible is spared. Electronic marks are placed, on the scan, on the upper and lower limits to be measured, and the unit will calculate the distance between the markers (see Figure 8.5). The orientation of the transducer can be marked on the scan, by the operator, to enable the viewer to relate the position of the scan to the patient.

Real time scanners are also used for determining the distance of the tumour from the surface of the patient, tumour volume, tumour relationship to vital structures and the position of the area marked on the patient relative to the tumour. The response of the treatment to the patient can be assessed, and it may be necessary to rearrange the treatment plan accordingly.[7]

An added advantage of ultrasound is that it is non-ionising at the levels used for imaging, so there are no untoward side-effects or genetic hazards. The hazards encountered with ultrasound, such as cavitation (bubble formation) and severe temperature rise, are generally at high power levels. It has been demonstrated that if the power levels do not go above 100 mW/cm^2, which is the case for imaging at present, there will be no adverse effects on tissue.

However, it is necessary to obtain plenty of experience in ultrasound scanning to be able to utilise the equipment efficiently, and interpret the scans accurately.

REFERENCES

1. Forster, E. (1985) *Equipment for Diagnostic Radiographers*, MTP Press, Lancaster, pp. 180-8.
2. Hussey, M. (1985) *Basic Physics and Technology of Medical Diagnostic Ultrasound*, Macmillan. London, pp. 17-22, 32-40.

3. Pickstock, B.T. [Mitsubishi Electric (UK) Ltd.] (1986) 'A digital video printer using thermal paper', *Electronic Technology*, **20**, 309-12.
4. Hussey, M. (1985) *Basic Physics of Diagnostic Ultrasound*, Macmillan, London, pp. 145-54.
5. McDicken, W.N. (1981) *Diagnostic Ultrasonics, Principles and Use of Instruments*, 2nd edn, John Wiley and Sons, Chichester, pp. 142-7, 187-207.
6. Lock, V. and Coules, D. (1986) 'Improved localisation for radical treatment of breast carcinoma using CT and Ultrasound', *Radiography*, **52**(606), 281-4.
7. Meire, H.B. and Farrant, P. (1982) *Basic Clinical Ultrasound*, British Institute of Radiology, Kent, pp. 137-42.

Private communications

D. Coules; L. Harvey; M. Lovegrove.

Manufacturers' literature

Agfa Gevaert, Scopix 100 The Grand Little Imager.
Computer Sonography Acuson 128.
Emisonic 4200 Nuclear Enterprises.
Fuji Film Thermal Imaging System.
Polaroid instant films in medical diagnostic imaging, Polaroid.
Siel, Vido Printer.
Shackman Super Seven Recording Camera, Shackman Instruments Ltd.
Toshiba, Sonolayer-L SAL-50A.
Ultrasound Static Scanning Unit type 1842, Bruel and Kjaer.
Ultramark 4 Ultrasound System, Scientific Medical Systems.

FURTHER READING

Bleehen, N.M., Glatstein, E. and Haybittle, J.L. (1983) *Radiation Therapy Planning*, Marcel Dekker, New York, pp. 99-103.
Curry, T.S., Dowdey, J.E., Murray Jr, R.C. (1984) *Christensen's Introduction to the Physics of Diagnostic Radiology*, 3rd edn, Lea and Febiger, Philadelphia, 351-400.
Goldberg, B.B. (1981) *Ultrasound in Cancer*, Churchill Livingstone, Edinburgh, pp. 167-85.
Kodak, 'Imaging via the cathode ray tube', *The Fundamentals of Radiographic Photography*, vol. IV, section 2.
Tiffany, R. (1978) *Oncology for Nurses and Health Care Professionals*, vol. 1, George Allen & Unwin Ltd, London, pp. 140-67.
Wells, P.N.T. (1982) *Scientific Basis of Medical Imaging*, Churchill Livingstone, Edinburgh, pp. 138-93.

9

Future Development — Magnetic Resonance Imaging (MRI)

The phenomenon of magnetic resonance was first described in 1946, but it was not until 1970 that the first magnetic resonance scanner was used clinically. This unit is still not a common piece of equipment because of the high cost of the scanner (£1–1.5 million).

A future development which is in the research phase at the present (according to Picker International Ltd) is to use magnetic resonance imaging as an aid for radiotherapy planning. The system would be similar to the way CT images are used with the radiotherapy planning computer (see Chapter 7).

The following text will give a simplified and brief outline of magnetic resonance imaging.

MRI SCANNER (see Figure 9.1)

The scanner used for magnetic resonance imaging consists of a large magnet, radiofrequency (RF) coils, gradient coils and computer system. There is also the couch which supports the patient inside the bore (aperture) of the magnet during the procedure.

The magnet

This is needed to produce a uniform and static external magnetic field, which will align the nuclei of atoms in the volume of the patient lying inside the magnet.

It is usually only the atoms with an odd number of nucleons (protons and neutrons) that align themselves in the direction of the magnetic field. This is because they produce their own magnetic field and act like tiny bar magnets. (Hydrogen, which is abundant in the form of water in the body, exhibits this property.) The effect of these small nuclear magnets is not

Figure 9.1: MRI scanner. (Courtesy of Picker International Ltd.)

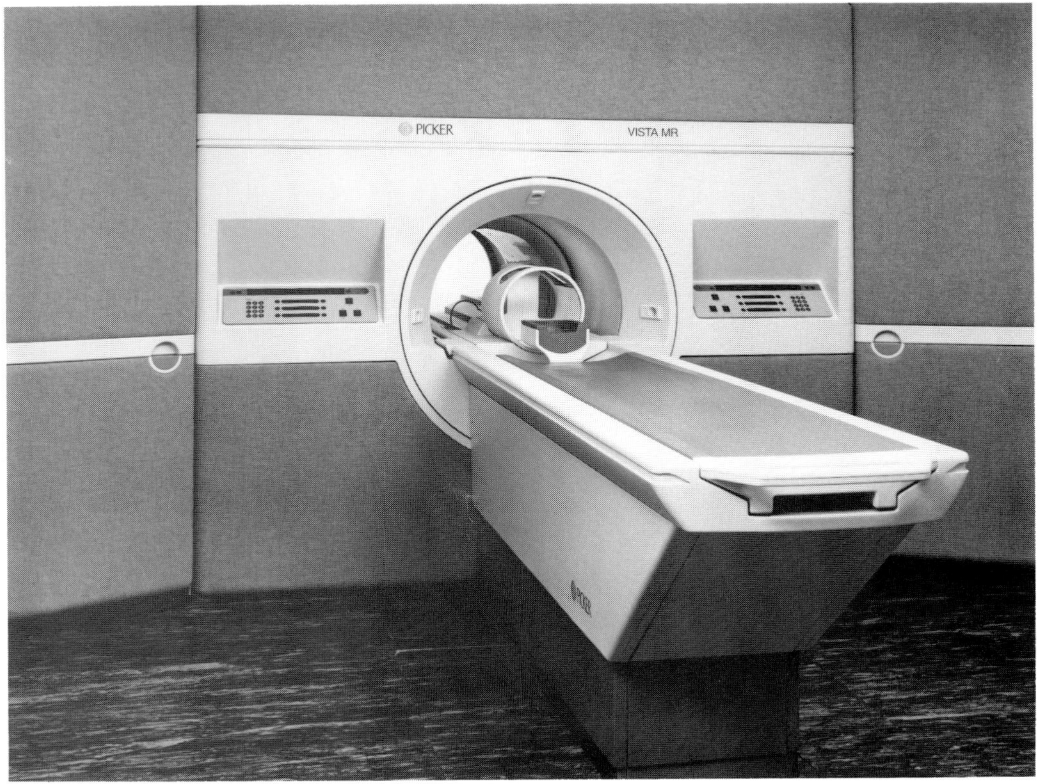

normally seen in tissue, as the magnetic fields are in random orientation and tend to cancel each other out. The nuclei of atoms with even numbers of nucleons generally do not produce a magnetic field.

An electromagnet of 0.1–0.3 tesla (unit of magnetic flux density) is commonly used for the scanner, but a more sophisticated unit may now have a magnet of 1.5–2.5 tesla. The magnet can weigh between three and five tonnes, be over 2 m high and 3 m long. It is usually placed inside a copper-screened room to eliminate RF interference from outside (see below). It is important the immediate vicinity contains no mobile ferrous metal objects as they will be instantly drawn towards the magnet. The magnet can be of two types, either superconductive or resistive.[1]

Superconductive magnet

This is wound with huge coils of conducting wire, made of niobium alloy or titanium alloy, which carry a current of electricity to produce a magnetic field. These coils have no electrical resistance at very low temperature so they are immersed in liquid helium (−269°C), in a container which is surrounded by liquid nitrogen (−200°C). The liquefied gases need constant replenishment because they evaporate into the atmosphere. When the coils are at the required temperature the current is supplied and will continue to flow around the coil without any further input of energy.

Resistive magnet

This usually has thick windings of copper or aluminium which carry the current to produce the magnetic field. The power needed to drive this current is between 30 and 40 kW, and produces a great deal of heat, so the coils are permanently cooled by water linked to a heat exchanger and pump. This is expensive, and a waste of heat unless it can be utilised.

Radiofrequency coils

The radiofrequency (RF) coils are shaped into curved panels which surround the patient during scanning. They act as a generator for RF excitation and as a receiver to detect the return signal.[1]

The RF signal which is generated is pulsed, and forms a magnetic field at 90° to the main magnetic field. This tilts the nuclei which are in alignment with the external magnetic field, and because they are spinning, the nuclei act like gyroscopes (spinning tops). They rotate around the direction of the main magnetic field while they slowly return to their original orientation. This action is called precession, and by rotating in this manner the bar magnets cause a current to flow in a detector coil, which acts like an aerial attached to a radiofrequency receiver. The signal is very small and is easily obscured by other RF noise from the environment, patient and coil. To maximise the detected signal the coil is placed as near as possible to the area being scanned, and often the coil is shaped to conform to body contours.

Gradient coils

To construct an image it is necessary to know where the signal originates with respect to the point of origin in the magnetic field. This is achieved by using gradient coils,[2] which produce an additional magnetic field which varies across the area being scanned. The frequency of the detected signal depends upon the strength of the magnetic field, and as this is now varied, depending on the signal frequency received it is possible to relate it to the area it has originated from. The gradient coils are usually mounted on or inside the main magnet.

Computer system

The image is formed by a specialised computer program being reconstructed in a similar fashion as for computed tomography (see Chapter 7). The digital image data are converted to an analogue signal so that the image can be viewed on a television monitor. The system for storage and making hard copies is the same as for CT images (see Chapter 7).

The images produced with the MRI scanner relate to the relaxation time, which is the time taken for the signal to disappear. There are two different types of relaxation times, T1 and T2, and they form the basis for contrast differences on the images.

T1, spin lattice relaxation time

This is defined as the time taken for the nuclei to return to their original alignment with the magnetic field. The extra energy from the RF pulse is lost into the surrounding lattice or environment. For soft tissue T1 can be 0.1–1 s.

T2 spin, spin relaxation time

After the RF pulse is applied the nuclei start to precess. However, they do not all precess at exactly the same rate, and they gradually get out of phase with each other. Their magnetic fields then cancel each other out and the signal disappears. The time taken for this to happen is called T2, and is shorter than the time for T1.

Hazard

As already mentioned, care must be taken with loose metal objects in the vicinity of the magnet as they can become projectiles, being drawn towards the magnet. Surgical clips in the patient may be dislodged, and the magnetic field will also affect a pacemaker used for cardiac disorders. Sensitive instruments such as cameras and watches may be damaged in the area of the magnetic field and any magnetic recording (tape, disk) will be erased.

The patient may also experience heating of tissue from the radio-frequency fields. The static magnetic field produces a current to flow in a moving conductor, for instance, blood, and the changing magnetic field produced by the gradient coils will produce a current in a static conductor, for example, a hip prosthesis. At present the above effects (heating and electromagnetic induction) are unconfirmed in clinical trials, and for the safe application of MRI the National Radiological Protection Board has proposed guidelines (for more information see Reference 2).

Figure 9.2: MRI scan — sagittal section (normal). (Courtesy of Picker International Ltd.)

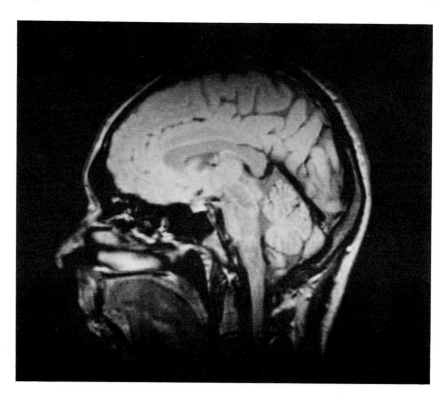

MRI FOR RADIOTHERAPY PLANNING

To be of value for radiotherapy planning it is important to be able to reproduce the treatment position during scanning and this, as with the CT scanner (see Chapter 7), is a slight problem for some areas.

At present rather large coils are placed in close proximity to the patient during scanning, so reproducing the position for some breast techniques, for example, with an arm pole protruding at right angles to the couch, would not be possible. Head immobilisation casts may also cause difficulties when scanning the head. These problems could be overcome in the future as it may be possible to place the patient on the outside of the magnet, rather than the inside, thus allowing easier positioning.

The benefit of being able to use the very detailed images (see Figures 9.2 and 9.3) produced with the MRI scanner for radiotherapy planning is that they show soft tissue with extremely good definition, and it is easier to differentiate between tumour and normal tissue.

Figure 9.3: MRI scan — transverse section showing metastases in the liver. (Courtesy of Picker International Ltd.)

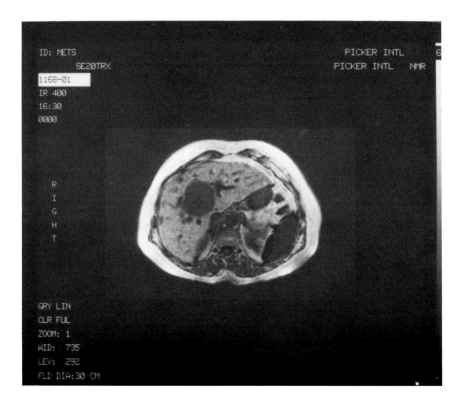

REFERENCES

1. Forster, E. (1985) *Equipment for Diagnostic Radiography*, MTP Press, Lancaster, pp. 212-14.
2. Picker International Ltd, *The Principles of NMR Imaging*, Technical Handbook, pp. 21, 37.

Private communication

Dr Delpy; Regional Centre for Radiotherapy and Oncology, Mount Vernon Hospital.

Manufacturers' literature

General Electric, Signa, Magnetic Resonance System.
Philips Medical Systems, Gyroscan, Magnetic Resonance Systems.

FURTHER READING

Chipperfield, S. (1984) 'Magnetic resonance imaging using a resistive system', *Radiography*, **50**(593), 213-19.
Curry, T.S., Dowdey, J.E. and Murray Jr, R.C. (1984) *Christensen's Introduction to the Physics of Diagnostic Radiology*, 3rd edn, Lea and Febiger, Philadelphia, pp. 461-503.
Kodak, 'Imaging via the cathode ray tube', *The Fundamentals of Radiographic Photography*, vol. IV, section 6.
Lerski, R.A. (1983) 'Physical principles of nuclear magnetic resonance imaging', *Radiography*, **49**(580), 85-90.
Thornton, M. (1984) 'An ABC of NMR', *Radiography*, **50**(593), 221-7.
Thornton, M. (1987) 'From NMR signal to MR image', *Radiography*, **53**(607), 31-43.

Index

£14-95